Audrey Eyton has spent most of her professional life working in the field of diet, nutrition and health, where she has become widely recognized and admired as a serious contributor and enlightened innovator. In 1969 she co-founded and directed the world's first magazine devoted to dieting, *Slimming Magazine*, and was responsible for many advances including the first low-fat slimming diet. In 1982 she published *The F-Plan Diet* which became an international multi-million-copy bestseller. Twenty-four years on she has written another ground-breaking book on diet and health, *The F2 Diet. The F2 Cookbook* is now available from Bantam Press. Audrey Eyton lives in Canterbury, Kent.

D0543605

# THE F2 DIET

## THE BIG BIO-BREAKTHROUGH

Audrey Eyton

**BANTAM BOOKS**

LONDON • TORONTO • SYDNEY • AUCKLAND • JOHANNESBURG

THE F2 DIET
A BANTAM BOOK : 9780553817522

Originally published in Great Britain by Bantam Press,
a division of Transworld Publishers

PRINTING HISTORY
Bantam Press edition published 2006
Bantam edition published 2007

1 3 5 7 9 10 8 6 4 2

Set in 11.25/14.5pt Minion by
Falcon Oast Graphic Art Ltd.

Bantam Books are published by Transworld Publishers,
61–63 Uxbridge Road, London W5 5SA,
a division of The Random House Group Ltd,
in Australia by Random House Australia (Pty) Ltd,
20 Alfred Street, Milsons Point, Sydney, NSW 2061, Australia,
in New Zealand by Random House New Zealand Ltd,
18 Poland Road, Glenfield, Auckland 10, New Zealand
and in South Africa by Random House (Pty) Ltd,
Isle of Houghton, Corner of Boundary Road & Carse O'Gowrie,
Houghton 2198, South Africa.

Printed and bound in Great Britain by
Cox & Wyman Ltd, Reading, Berkshire.

Papers used by Transworld Publishers are natural, recyclable
products made from wood grown in sustainable forests. The
manufacturing processes conform to the environmental
regulations of the country of origin.

# THE F2 DIET

# Acknowledgements

Many people have contributed to The **F2 Diet** and to all of them I am deeply grateful. Dr Alison Stephen, the distinguished Cambridge nutrition scientist, was a fount of information and an exacting taskmaster – fiercely determined that I should get scientific facts correct. Any mistakes that might have crept in are entirely due to me and not to her. She will make me suffer for them!

I am also grateful for time and information generously given by Dr Sheila Bingham, Deputy Director of the MRC Dunn Human Nutrition Unit at Cambridge; to two close friends of mine, Professor Philip James, Chairman of the International Obesity Task Force, and Professor Catherine Geissler of King's College, London University; to Dr Tony Leeds, also of King's, London; Dr Susan Jebb of MRC Human Nutrition Research, Cambridge; Professor David Southgate; Dr John Cummings; and Dr Ken Heaton.

It was a delight to work again with a valued long-time colleague, home economist Glynis McGuinness, who has an iron determination to get her nutritional figures exact, down to that of the last grain of rice. She was responsible for all Fat and Calorie Controller figures, and cookery expert Maggie Pannell for the F2 recipes.

Peter Cox has been a valued collaborator and sounding board as well as my agent.

Lastly I am grateful to all my friends for their encouragement and support, and to the memory of Matthew, my total inspiration in everything I try to do.

*Scientific Consultant*, Dr Alison Stephen
*Home Economist*, Glynis McGuinness
*Realistic Recipes*, Maggie Pannell

# Introduction

## F2 in action – now comes the proof!

UNBEATABLE FOR FAST WEIGHT LOSS, able to make you feel fitter in days, The **F2 Diet** resulted from three years intensive research at the cutting edge centres of nutritional science.

For me that was the hard part – now comes the fun: seeing **F2**'s advanced formula in action, discovering how many different weight and health problems it has already solved in recent months:

### Weight-gain problem solved!

Mary Clark, for instance, was worried about the surplus stone which had crept on over the past three years. Like her friend Ruth Arnold, and many others I've heard from, it took her just a month to polish it off with **F2**. Inspired and surprised she's gone on to shed another stone and is still losing.

Mary and Ruth weren't aiming at 'size 8', but, rightly realised the more you gain the easier it is to gain more – even reach the point of no return. Almost inevitable, in fact, unless you take decisive action. Mary and Ruth did. And **F2**, with its inbuilt fast-loss factor, did it for them, reversing their gains in record time.

### Time problem solved!

● Radio presenter and disc-jockey Andy Walker knew he needed 'to get off the fast-food track'.

Working erratic hours, getting home too tired to cook, turned him into McDonald's man. From work-friendly **F2** Andy discovered that fast meals needn't be fattening.

Low-cal stir-fries, for example, can be cooked in minutes with veg bought ready chopped and well chosen low-fat sauces (see guide on page 157). Now lean, fit and trimmed of 18 surplus pounds in weeks, Andy found losing weight no hassle. **F2** fit into his fast and busy life.

## 'Inside' problem solved!

● Lythe, lean, and lovely yoga teacher Cheryl Rivers already had a perfect figure. But, along with half the British population, many of them young and slim, she'd had a life-long 'loo-problem' – solved in days (see Chapter 4) when she started eating the **F2** way.

'The **F2 Diet** was a complete revelation,' says Cheryl. 'It cleared and detoxed my system, banished that bloated feeling in 48 hours, got my insides working properly for the first time in my life.'

Now it's Cheryl's bible. Her sister, husband, father, best friend, best friend's husband have all been converted and Cheryl feels as wonderful as she looks.

## Health problem solved!

● Cheryl's best friend Ann Neal did have a weight problem and with it, like so many others, threatening signals of ill-health. Now with weight down nearly 2 stone, and cholesterol and blood-pressure reaching healthier levels she feels better than she's felt for years.

Says Ann: 'I faced up to the fact that there's no such thing as a free lunch where health is concerned. Medical drugs and operations all have their downside. **F2** proved to me that it's what you eat for lunch (and dinner) that really makes the difference. Why eat yourself ill when it's surprisingly easy to eat yourself slim and fit?'

## Plateau problem solved!

● After losing two stone over a year bride-to-be Catrina Bulbeck had reached a weight-loss 'plateau'. Just couldn't budge another pound in time for her wedding, whatever she did – until she tried **F2**.

After long periods of dieting the body tends to use less calories, and final surplus pounds can become stubborn. The **F2 Diet**, which helpfully 'wastes' some of the calories consumed (see Chapter 5) got Catrina's weight dropping again – just in time. The week before her wedding she reached her goal and took her wedding dress in for 'tucks'. Bridegroom, schoolteacher Dave Chaplin, who dieted with her, also weighed half a stone less when they stepped lightly down the aisle.

## Temptation problem solved!

● Nurse Lorna Jones believed she was a chocoholic, but found she barely gave chocs a thought as she watched her weight bump down by more than 20 lbs on The **F2 Diet**.

'I found the plan an inspiration,' wrote Lorna, 'It's become almost second nature. I love the foods and the recipes – which don't assume you're cooking for an army! My food tastes are changing. I've even learned to love beans which I came to hate at an over-strict school. My daughter, a scientist, is also living the **F2** way and says she can't fault its approach. All my other diet books are going off to the charity shop.'

## Will-power problem solved!

● Like most dieters, clinical secretary Sue Perkins wondered whether she'd have the will-power to lose weight. On The **F2 Diet**, she found she didn't need any.

'I loved eating the **F2** way, it was no hardship – a pleasure.

Losing a surplus stone just seemed like a bonus,' said Sue. 'It was genuinely effortless for me and made me feel fantastic, heaps better. I have loads of energy and people keep telling me how much younger I look.'

## Motivational problem solved!

● Doctor's receptionist Susan Coomb needed motivating to shed weight.

'Someone sent me a copy of The **F2 Diet**, I read it and that did it,' says Susan. 'For the first time I took on board the fact that I was probably killing myself with the surplus weight I'd been carrying for 20 years. I liked the look of the uncomplicated **F2** meals, got going and was amazed at how easy it is. I don't feel hungry, I feel full and the weight is rolling off – a stone to date. I'm actually enjoying the food and think I've become addicted to Tex Mex Soup (page 111). Wish I'd realized 20 years ago that dieting needn't be difficult – but better late than never.'

## Your problems solved!

● Whatever your weight or health problem, turn to page 18 and discover what **F2** can do for you. It's the new route to a new you – the one that does the lot for weight, looks and health. Nothing is more likely to zap off your weight and zip up your life. Read on and revolutionize the way your whole body looks and works.

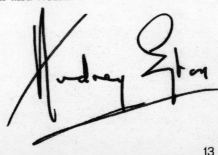

PART

1

# WHAT F2 CAN DO FOR YOU

# 1

# THE BAD NEWS AND THE GOOD NEWS

# What F2 can do for you

➤ **Remove your surplus fat at a faster rate than any other diet** of the same calorie intake.

➤ **Enable you to lose weight** without feeling hungry.

➤ **Mobilize an 'army' of good bacteria** to boost your feel-good factor and help protect you against cancers.

➤ **Rejuvenate and revitalize** your inner health.

➤ **Speed away health-threatening waste matter** which can linger dangerously in your colon for days.

➤ **Lower your cholesterol** to protect your heart.

➤ **Slow the release of sugar into your blood** to prevent 'rebound hunger' and health risks.

➤ **Feed your brain with the nourishment it needs** to maximize thinking ability and your body with a multitude of health-promoting nutrients.

B RACE YOURSELF, I think we'd better start with the bad news. Think of this as 'tough love'. If you are overweight you are at high risk of cancers of the colon, breast and – in the case of men – the prostate. Your heart is under serious threat. You are a prime candidate for diabetes. Oh, and add hypertension and strokes to your risk list.

Your arteries are almost certainly dangerously clogged with cholesterol. Bad bacteria are busy doing very nasty things inside your gut. And as for the toxic, cancer-causing waste matter which has been lingering in your colon for days, let's not even go there. *Well, at least for the present . . .*

But here is the good news. By changing your diet you can shed all your surplus fat at maximum speed and at the same time dramatically reduce your risk of all those health threats and many more. You can start to feel good *from inside* – better than you have ever felt. Your blood will begin to flow freely through your arteries and all that colon-clogging waste matter will be speeded away. A mighty army of good bacteria will go to work in your insides like Dyno-Rod. You will actually experience the proof of that within days. And while they're at it they will also act in a multitude of other ways to rejuvenate your system and restore the bio-balance essential for positive health.

**But you must choose the right diet to achieve all these benefits.**

Any slimming diet can get you slim if you can keep to it. All are simply ways of reducing calorie intake to force your body to consume its own surplus fat. This, apart from increasing calorie output by exercise, is the only weight-loss method known to science.

But many slimming diets, particularly the low-carbohydrate crop of recent years, won't achieve those vital inner-health changes. In the long term their effect is likely to be quite the reverse. They are leading you even further in the wrong direction, making matters even worse. You are unlikely to suffer the dangerous consequences in weeks or even months, and may experience temporary well-being from shedding weight. But, as many millions of others have already discovered to their cost, this pattern of eating will catch up with you eventually.

That's why so many nutritional scientists so strongly cautioned against the low-carbohydrate dieting craze, which has left some dangerously confused ideas in its wake.

So what diets do the *real* experts recommend for weight loss? Or for health and looks? Happily, contrary to commonplace myths, there isn't one good diet for cancer prevention, another for heart health or diabetes prevention, nor for that matter different diets to improve your skin, hair, teeth, increase your energy, sharpen your mind, lift your mood.

There is one good diet that does the lot and, at the same time, removes fat at maximum speed.

Unlike many other diets – those low-carb diets in particular – it works beneficially deep in your insides as it dissolves your visible bulges. It gets good bacteria working for you in many different ways. It speeds away dangerous colon and artery clogging matter as it speeds away the pounds.

There are two reasons why surplus weight is dangerous. Just carrying it around puts internal organs under strain.

And those foods largely responsible for making people fat also happen to be mainly responsible for life-threatening illnesses and generally sluggish states of incipient ill health. There is evidence of this in population studies from all over the world. Truck-loads of evidence. Ship-loads of evidence. Whole convoys of ship-loads of evidence.

There is just as much evidence, much of it recent and from irrefutable major studies, that the foods you will eat in increasing quantity on **F2** have just the opposite effect. They are the good guys, the protective army that will storm through your system. Think of them as the SOS – Save Our System – platoon. Time to call them into action.

## Why follow a health-suspect slimming diet when, without any additional effort, you could lose surplus fat more speedily on a diet that can vastly improve your health?

I too have read the other diet books and very convincing many of them were too. If Nobel Prizes were awarded for salesmanship I would, at one time, have personally nominated the late Dr Atkins and his spin doctors who sold the world such staggering quantities of books, nutritional supplements, drinks, cereals, soup mixes – even birthday cakes and cruises – in an unparalleled diet-marketing operation before their fortunes declined. They could certainly have sold me double-glazing. But a diet? I don't think so. Having supervised hundreds of people on low-carb diets myself, I wasn't in the market for miracle-myths in that department.

I too could boast of decades of experience in so many areas of weight control: personally helping hundreds to lose weight, collaborating with the world's leading obesity experts, founding the first diet magazine, writing a best-selling diet, helping to establish health farms, slimming clubs . . . But despite all that, I could still be trying to sell you my own crackpot theory. Even a well-meant, deeply believed but nevertheless dubious, even dangerous theory.

Even the most intelligent people are gullible when it comes to diets. Wishful thinking too often prevails. It is exceedingly hard to recognize what's rot and what's not. Who to believe and who not to. That is why I must caution you even against believing me.

Wouldn't it be wonderful if we could get together, say, a hundred of the world's leading experts and ask them what really is the most effective diet for weight loss and health?

*Well, hang on in there, maybe we can . . .*

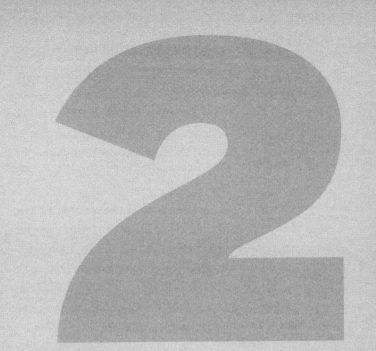

# 2

# THE
# GOOD-CARB
# COME-BACK

YOU COULD HAVE knocked me down with a celery stick when I learned, a few years ago, that the old low-carbohydrate diet was back. Been there, done that, while most of you were still being spoon-fed strained carrots.

Way back in the sixties, in the UK at least, it was just about the only known way to diet. You cut out those 'naughty' carbs like potatoes, bread, porridge, rice, pasta and breakfast cereals as well as puds, pastry and chocolates. So naturally, when I became Beauty Editor of Britain's biggest selling women's magazine, that was the route I took.

I saw people losing weight on such diets – at least for a while, until weight loss often plateaued-out – for some perfectly obvious reasons. Alcohol and sugary drinks were banned. That, in itself, substantially cuts calorie intake for most. Low-carb diets limit variety of food, which tends to make you eat less – no puds allowed, for instance, to tempt your taste buds with sweetness, however full your tum. More crucially, low-carb diets cut out the very many foods such as cake, biscuits, pastry, pies, puds, chips, chocolate, dairy ice-creams, pizzas in which carbohydrates hang out with a fat friend – a highly undesirable companion called fat.

When you cut out carbs you also cut out calories in the fats normally eaten with them.

More than twice as high in calories as any other food, fat is the real demon king of the dieting firmament. Always has been, still is. The quantity of fat you eat is the major dietary determinant of whether you are fat or slim. This isn't a matter of theories or debate – it is simply and irrefutably a matter of maths:

One gram carbohydrate or protein = **4 calories**

One gram fat = **9 calories**

# YOU CAN'T ARGUE WITH THAT!

But there were ways in which people still ate more fat than was good for them on those old-fashioned low-carb diets and – here's what particularly worried the experts – this was largely health-threatening, cholesterol-raising, saturated fat. Dangerous fat. You get particularly large quantities of this in dairy products such as cheese, butter and cream and a good deal from meat dishes.

Happily the factors that helped some people shed weight on low-carb diets were those that also led most of them to shed the diet itself sooner or later. Monotony set in. It's all very well to be told (unwisely) that you can gorge on meat and cheese, but what if you are yearning for something different? And, as it turns out, often something that would be far more healthy to eat.

'A significant proportion of the population consumes less than the recommended amount of fruit and vegetables and fibre but more than the recommended amount of fat, saturated fat, salt and sugar. Such poor nutrition is a major cause of ill health and premature death.'

UK DEPARTMENT OF HEALTH, 2005

Fortunately, fad, fashion and dieters have moved on and are beginning to realize that some carbohydrate-rich foods are not only good for health, they are the most helpful foods you can eat if you want to lose weight. Even more valuable, as you will discover from new evidence in this book, than was previously realized. So it's just as well that fashion is beginning to follow where science has led ...

## Globesity – the shock that shook the diet world

Half a century ago, the belief prevailed among nutritionists that lots of animal protein and dairy products were a good thing. You just couldn't get too much of them. Or so they thought until nasty things started happening to those in affluent countries eating such foods in ever-increasing quantities. Slowly ... steadily ... and then explosively it became evident that certain deadly ailments were increasing to epidemic proportions. Cancers of the colon,

'Diets rich in dietary fibre have been shown to have a number of beneficial effects, including decreased risk of coronary heart disease and improvement in laxation . . . Making fibre-rich food choices more often is likely to confer significant health benefits.'

DIETARY GUIDELINES FOR AMERICANS 2005,
US DEPARTMENT OF HEALTH AND HUMAN SERVICES

breast and prostate and coronary heart disease were fast becoming – and have now become – the predominant causes of premature death in the West. But people in the developing world, still living on traditional plant-based diets, remained free of these degenerative ailments. Until, that is, our fast-food giants moved in.

Today there is a worldwide epidemic known to the alarmed world of nutritional science as 'globesity'. Here's what's happening. In countries in what is called 'nutritional transition', rural communities continue to eat traditional diets. Though still prey to many of the infectious diseases which we've got sorted in the West, our weight and health problems remain relatively unknown to them. They remain slim even when food is plentiful. But the increasing numbers flooding into cities and influenced by our diet are piling into burgers, fried chicken, pizzas and other animal-based products. And, among these people, the incidence of obesity and Western cancers and coronaries is absolutely soaring.

## Risks – the real extent

Few people fully realize the mega-risks they run on a typical Western diet in terms of cancers alone. Scientists don't help when they simply state that 30 to 35 per cent of cancers are diet-related. In this they include, for instance, lung cancer, mainly caused by smoking, and skin cancer, mainly caused by overexposure to the sun. But when it comes to those all-too-common cancers of the colon, breast and prostate, the dietary link is much, much, much stronger. As it is with heart disease.

---

# CHEW ON THESE FACTS:

An American is **TWENTY** times more likely to get colon cancer than is a vegetarian Asian. He is **SEVENTEEN** times more likely to get heart disease than is a rural Chinese.

---

So let's consider what people who don't risk our killer diseases and obesity are chewing to protect themselves and what they aren't chewing to cause such dangers. And what exactly is going on in their insides. And whether, without going to extremes, we can adjust our Western diets to gain their advantages.

The main foods they *aren't* eating frequently and in quantity are dairy products and meat. Most of us eat more of these foods in a day than they eat in a week or more. For many of them, meat is a treat – a garnish – and dairy products simply aren't consumed at all.

Mostly they are living on high-carbohydrate diets based on staples such as rice, maize (corn), millet or wheat-based foods such as bread and noodles, and on vegetables and seasonally available fruit. In doing so they are consuming very large quantities of substances which protect against Western diseases. Have you noticed that whenever new research reveals a protective nutrient, whether for eyes, heart, colon, kidneys, arteries, brain, even virility, it is, almost invariably, a substance found in plants?

## Why food works – not pills, capsules and other supplements

The protective substances in plant foods can't simply be consumed in the form of supplements. These substances are highly complex. Some of them interact with each other and they can only work to their full beneficial effect when consumed in the form of a variety of foods.

Among them is one particular substance which is, in itself, of great complexity and known to benefit our health in a multiplicity of ways. That is why just about every government and publicly funded health organization throughout the Western world highly recommends that most of us double – yes, double – our present intake. This substance is known as dietary fibre. It is found only in fruit, vegetables and grain-based cereal foods which have not been overprocessed. Most of it is the cell-wall material of such foods.

Dietary fibre is so beneficial in weight control that people who eat enough of it simply don't get fat. But before I tell you more, I did hint at calling in one hundred of the world's leading experts to advise you on your weight. Happily, I am able to do so courtesy of the United Nations' authority on health, the World Health Organization. Alarmed by galloping globesity, the WHO asked more than one hundred top experts from all over the world to confer. They worked at it for two years. The summing up of their conclusions:

'The promotion of healthy diets that are low in fat, high in complex carbohydrates and contain large amounts of fresh fruit and vegetables should be a priority in obesity prevention.'

But why stop at consulting only one hundred world experts when the advice of literally thousands is available? The WHO's dietary recommendations are in line with those of all major government and public-funded organizations concerned with Western diet-related diseases. Much as mavericks love to chafe against the view of the vast majority (I have been known to veer in that direction myself), there are occasions on which the vast majority are right. This is one of them. The evidence in their support is just too huge, too overwhelming and it keeps on mounting. I'd stake my life on them being right. I do, in what I choose to eat.

It's obvious why experts give the thumbs down to fats. Their calorie content is mega-high and saturated fat is Culprit Number One in clogging the arteries with heart-threatening cholesterol. But to understand more fully their emphasis on eating more plant-based foods, come with me on a revealing little canter around your colon. It's high time you actually saw what is going on in your insides.

# Look what's going on inside your colon on a typical western high-protein diet!

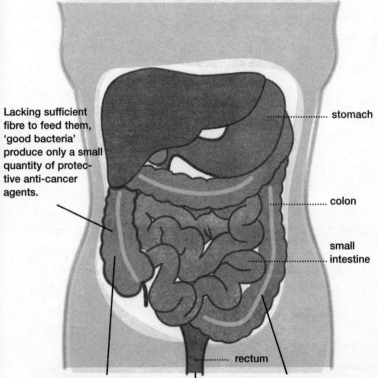

Lacking sufficient fibre to feed them, 'good bacteria' produce only a small quantity of protective anti-cancer agents.

stomach

colon

small intestine

rectum

Fed mainly on protein, 'bad bacteria' thrive here producing a large quantity of ammonia and nitrogen compounds suspected of causing cancer. Substances in red and processed meats are particularly highly suspect.

In the high powered 'drying machine' on this side of the colon, waste matter, already low in volume, becomes dryer, firmer and resistant to onward movement. Food residues, high in carcinogens, linger in dangerous contact with the gut wall for days.

## It takes from three days to a week for all the waste matter from food consumed to be expelled in the faeces.

31

# Now see what's going on inside on a fibre-rich plant-based diet.

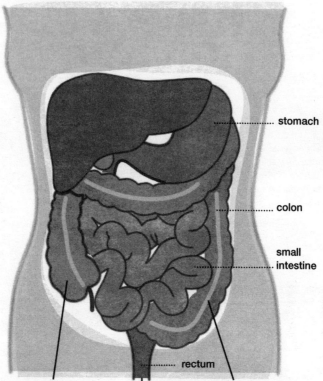

stomach

colon

small intestine

rectum

'Good bacteria' feed on fibre which stimulates them to increase in number. In doing so they *reduce* cancer-causing substances such as ammonia and *increase* protective anti-cancer agents.

Bulked and diluted by water held in undigested fibre and in 'good bacteria', waste matter is speeded through the colon. Cancer-causing substances are not allowed to linger in dangerous contact with the gut wall.

**Waste matter is expelled effortlessly, usually within one and a half days of food being eaten. Some calories are expelled undigested, giving a weight loss advantage.**

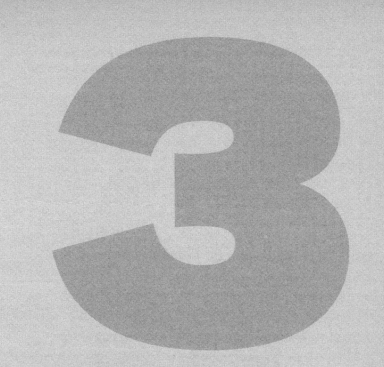

# TIME TO
# GET THINGS
# MOVING

WHO WOULD have thought that colonic irrigation, once considered the eccentric practice of old maids, would become sexy? But where Princess Di led other trend-setters followed. Now, in certain circles, it has become as routine as a bikini-line wax.

Just a passing fad? Maybe so. But behind it lies an instinct dating back more than a hundred years: a sense that nasty toxic substances are collecting in your colon, threatening your health and making you feel not so good in general. So strong was this belief late in the nineteenth century that some surgeons actually removed perfectly normal colons in the belief that this would make people feel better.

Leap forward a century or so and guess what? Scientists are now convinced that nasty toxic substances are indeed collecting in many people's colons, although they wouldn't exactly put it in those words. They would speak, rather, of carcinogens – substances implicated in causing cancer. In the world's great nutritional divide, it is the colons of those following typical high-animal-protein Western diets that are giving serious cause for concern. And it isn't a matter of the medical world 'holding its breath' for the outcome. The outcome is already evident in the explosion of Western cancers and other degenerative diseases.

It's all happening – now!

The fact that high-fibre diets offer major health benefits in this and other respects has been known to science for years. But two decades of research since I wrote the high-fibre F-Plan Diet have:

➤ **Shed** new light and more emphasis on how and why this eating pattern is crucial for health.

➤ **Emphasized** that quantity of dietary fibre isn't all that counts: equally important is 'diversity' – getting different forms of fibre from all three sources: vegetables, grains and fruit.

➤ **Revealed** how, by choosing fibre-rich foods in the right form and physical structure, you can make them even more effective and protective.

➤ **Discovered** – in cutting-edge science – that substances called 'resistant starch' and 'oligosaccharides', which are now considered components of dietary fibre, play a vital role in cancer prevention and other aspects of health.

Most dramatically and excitingly, what has emerged in recent research is evidence of a life-or-death battle (it can be as crucial as that!) going on inside your intestine right now: bacteria wars.

It sounds like science fiction. Remarkably, it is science fact. Inside your colon are two colonies of bacteria – good bacteria protecting your health, bad bacteria seriously threatening it. If you haven't done so already, I urge you to study the illustrations on pages 31 and 32 to see what is going on and why.

Which army prevails depends on the type of food you put in your mouth. Wolf down a lot of meat and that which reaches the colon feeds the bad bacteria, stimulating them to produce toxic substances suspected of causing cancer. Eat, instead, a diet rich in vegetables, pulses and grain-based foods which haven't been over-processed and you feed the good bacteria, causing them to increase in number and produce substances that protect your health in many ways as well as speeding away the dangerous substances. New research suggests they may protect against infectious illnesses, possibly even colds and flu, as well as degenerative diseases such as colon and breast cancers.

Speed counts where the functions of the colon are concerned. The colonic-irrigation crew are at least right in sensing that. Modern scientific techniques that can track food through the body reveal that, on a Western diet, it can take up to a week for the contents of a whole meal to pass through the system.

So it can be 'Hello again' to the remains of last Monday's bacon and eggs when you visit the bathroom a week later, and, hanging around in there feeding bad bacteria, they really haven't been doing you any good turns.

# BACTERIA
## meet (and feed) the elite!

Research on the health impact of good bacteria has revealed a particular type of ultra-good bacteria – bifidobacteria. These are emerging as the top task force among health protectors.

Bifidobacteria feed and flourish on a component of dietary fibre called oligosaccharides, only present in certain foods. The onion family – onions, shallots and leeks – are the best food sources, along with asparagus, chicory and artichokes. Some is also present in wheat, oats, bananas and pulses. Although garlic is a rich source, its pungent flavour prevents it from being eaten in sufficient quantity to be of much use in this respect, while wheat, though a less concentrated source of oligosaccharides, is also of value because it is eaten in larger volume.

Bifidobacteria have become a major focus of scientific interest. They play a key role in the bacteria wars by producing substances which can kill off some of the bad bacteria. They are also thought to help prevent harmful substances being absorbed by the colon lining and to protect against infections in this way.

Human breast milk is another source of oligosaccharides. In this scientists suspect they have at last discovered the reason why it tends to prove more protective to infants than formula milk.

Today our bacterial balance is threatened as never before. Travel can expose us to new strains of bacteria, harmless to overseas populations adapted to them but potentially harmful to us. Antibiotics, taken to kill off harmful germs, also destroy good bacteria, leaving the gut more vulnerable to bad bacteria. Antibiotic and drug residues in factory-farmed meat and in seafood and the long-lasting side-effects of medical drugs can have similar detrimental effects. And, paradoxically, our modern emphasis on hygiene leaves us less resistant to those bad bacteria which do succeed in reaching our systems. All such factors accelerate the tendency for the number of good bacteria in the gut to diminish as we age and healthy bioactivity to slow down.

To restore and rejuvenate the health of your colon, where much of your immune system is located, there are two things you need to do for it every day. One is to ensure that it becomes populated with an army of good bacteria. The other is to ensure that it expels waste matter fast. And only the right kind of diet will do both. There aren't any short cuts.

## Good bacteria yogurts like Yakult and Actimel?

These increasingly popular products are soundly based on science. Those known as probiotics contain good bacteria to add to those in your colon. Once there, however, these bacteria cannot thrive and survive for long without a plentiful and regular supply of the food they need. That food is the non-digestible ingredients in fibre-rich plants which reach the colon intact. Fed with a generous quantity of dietary fibre, the good bacteria multiply, and so do their health benefits. So these products (even those which contain 'prebiotics', which help to feed good bacteria) only offer their full benefit as part of the right diet.

## Colonic irrigation?

In flushing out the bad bacteria and waste matter lingering in the colon this does a good job. But here's the snag. It flushes out the good bacteria at the same time. And scientists are more and more convinced that a girl's (or boy's) best friends are good bacteria. Hence, unless there are special medical reasons, frequent colonic irrigation is not encouraged.

## Drinking lots of water?

It's a logical idea that drinking lots of water will flush out the toxins from your system. Pity it doesn't work like that. Unless you are eating the right diet to 'hold' and utilize that water, the excess achieves no particular benefit.

The left-hand side of your colon contains a drying machine worthy of a Bosch or Bendix lifetime warranty. It dries up waste matter with remarkable speed and efficiency. This is not good news for those on high-protein low-fibre diets. Dried-out waste matter cannot slide on easily through the colon, as waste matter should. Its onward progress can be slowed down for days.

In contrast, on a plant-based high-fibre diet, two beneficial things occur. The large colony of good bacteria you've built up absorb a large quantity of liquid. These bacteria actually consist of 80 per cent water. At the same time the non-fermented fibre from your diet is also holding water like a sponge. And your bodily Bosch or Bendix can't dry out water when it is held inside bacteria or fibre. Hence waste matter remains soft and bulky, rather than dry, and easily and effortlessly speeds onwards.

So, given that you drink sufficient (at least two litres a day in total liquids), it's not how much you drink that makes the difference. It's what you eat that determines the effectiveness of what you drink in 'cleaning out your system'.

## Fibre supplements

Sorry, there really are no shortcuts. If you hope that taking a fibre supplement while following a low-carb diet will do all that's necessary you've forgotten that protein in red and processed meat is feeding bad bacteria. Chomping away on it, they are producing some pretty dangerous substances in your gut. But that isn't the half of it.

Dietary fibre is a highly complex substance. It is present in varying quantities in all fruits, vegetables and grain-based foods, although it has been mostly stripped out of highly refined foods such as sugar, white flour and white rice.

The fibre in fruit is different from the fibre in vegetables, which in turn is different from the fibre in grains. What's more, the type of fibre in any specific fruit differs to some extent from that in any other type of fruit. Ditto vegetables and grains.

These different forms of fibre offer different health benefits. For instance, that in fruit and veg is particularly beneficial in stimulating the growth of good bacteria. The fibre in pulses is also so effective in lowering so-called 'bad cholesterol' in the bloodstream that this alone would be a good enough reason for eating a high-fibre diet.

But it is the fibre in some grains, acting like a sponge, holding water and bulking out colon contents, which most impacts on transit time – speeding away waste matter. Wheat fibre is outstanding in this respect. Much more effective than any other food.

'Scientists are now convinced that nasty toxic substances are indeed collecting in many people's colons.'

When you eat fibre in food, rather than supplements, you also gain major benefits from other substances associated with it. One of these is starch, a once-despised component of carbohydrate. Some starch – 'resistant starch' as it is called – passes through to the colon undigested. Recent studies reveal it to be a favourite food of good bacteria, more effective than anything else in stimulating them to produce a powerful anti-cancer agent called butyrate and in suppressing cancer-causing ammonia.

Bananas, when eaten when their skin is still a little green, are a particularly rich source of resistant starch. So, oddly enough, are certain carbohydrates which scientists refer to as 'retrograded' – those which are cooked then eaten cold. Cold pasta and cold potatoes are our most common sources.

Wheat fibre helps to push more resistant starch right through the colon to protect it end to end. This is just one example of how beneficial substances from different foods interact to produce a multiplicity of health benefits.

Many more benefits no doubt remain to be discovered, because what is known is this: it is the diets rich in a variety of *foods* (not supplements) containing fibre which really deliver on health protection not only in your colon but throughout your whole system. A growing body of scientific evidence suggests that fibre helps protect against breast cancer by reducing levels of oestrogen hormones circulating in the body and fosters bone health by increasing calcium absorption. These foods are also simply loaded with minerals, vitamins and other health-protecting nutrients.

By now, chatting so intimately about your colon, I trust we've become friends. I hope so, because now I'm about to ask you to come with me to the smallest room.

# 4

# PRIVATE BUT IMPORTANT

NOW LET'S ALL be grown-up about this. In an age when sexual perversions are served up on mainstream TV and scenes of explicit violence make softies like me long to hide behind cinema seats whimpering 'I want my Mummy!', we are about to discuss the one remaining unmentionable: human excrement.

And we'll discuss this in detail, even view illustrations – shock, horror – for some very sound reasons.

For your health's sake, it is vitally important that the waste matter from the food you eat has a fast transit time through your colon. But here's the tricky part: just because you have a daily bowel movement you can't assume your transit time is quick. What is being excreted today could be the waste matter from the food you ate last week.

Neither, you'll appreciate, have we any way to compare our bowel movements with those of others. The Germans, I'm told, have 'viewing platforms' down their loos. Good for the Germans. But this still doesn't provide an opportunity for comparisons (we trust!). Hence, most people assume their bowel function is normal and healthy, when, in fact, on a Western diet, all too often it isn't. And that 'all too often' applies equally to young and old.

Modern research refutes the idea that slow transit time and constipation are only experienced by the elderly. Young women, indeed most women of child-bearing age, are particularly prone to this problem. Little wonder that Mick Jagger's daughter Lizzy was reportedly put off modelling mainly because 'all the girls are in the loos all the time . . . completely constipated'. Studies suggest, in fact, that only a minority of the British and those on similar diets are functioning healthily in the colonic department. Which helps to account for our particularly high cancer rates.

## So how can you tell whether your transit time is sufficiently fast?

Well, for starters, you've certainly got problems if you take a newspaper, book, or radio to while away your time on the loo. Bathroom libraries are a terrible testimony to widespread Western bowel dysfunction. As, heaven preserve us, are those loo-side telephones in US hotels!

**Ease, speed and effortlessness** are an essential element in a healthy bowel movement. You should have to strain no more to empty your bowels than to empty your bladder. And the process should be almost as quick.

**Regularity,** although it doesn't automatically guarantee that transit time is fast, will happen automatically when transit time speeds up. If you are in otherwise normal health (and not on some medical drugs which can cause constipation), expect an effortless bowel movement at least once a day, maybe more frequently, when you switch to

**F2**. But have no fear, this won't have the liquid consistency and socially embarrassing urgency of diarrhoea.

**Colour** is a very important clue. Diluted by the water in good bacteria and fibre, a healthy bowel movement will be light brown as opposed to dark brown. It will be bulky and generally large in volume, rather than what one scientist described as 'joined-up rabbit pellets'.

'Just because you have a daily bowel movement you can't assume your transit time is fast.'

**'Floaters'** are good news. Although this will depend, to a degree, on what types of fibre-rich foods you ate on the previous day, it is true what they say about sinkers and floaters. Faeces from fibre-rich diets usually float. More flushing may be required, but it's a small price to pay.

**Food particles** are good news too. For those prepared to peer even more closely into the matter, little particles of undigested food such as sweetcorn, bits of greenery and beans are often detectable in the healthy faeces from a high-fibre diet.

'Most people assume their bowel movement is normal and healthy when, on a Western diet, all too often it isn't.'

Anyway, you can not only see the difference on the following pages, you can experience it for yourself within a few days when you start **F2**. Because most people in the

West eat so little fibre, I've suggested that you step up wheat fibre (the best 'fast forward' for transit time) gradually for the first few days to allow your body to adjust. During that period you'll still be clearing away the dry, hard-to-shift waste matter clogging your colon from previous meals. But then, increasingly, you will really start to experience the difference a healthy diet can make and understand that what you thought was normal and healthy wasn't.

But what about your weight loss? Turn to the next chapter, we're getting there . . .

# VIEW FROM THE LOO

These illustrations, adapted from the Bristol Stool Form Scale by kind permission of bowel expert Dr Ken Heaton, can help you recognize, from the stools you pass, whether things are really going right in your insides. The morning bowel movement tends to be the best by which to judge.

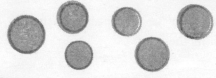

**Type 1** Separate hard lumps like nuts.
You've really got problems. Stools like this are usually hard to pass and strongly indicate a slow transit time. After a bowel movement of this nature you are likely to sense that all waste matter has not been fully evacuated; some of it remains inside.

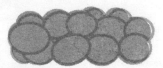

**Type 2** Sausage-like but lumpy.
A joined-up version of Type 1 and almost as unhealthy, for the same reasons. This type is very common on a typical Western diet which is too high in animal products and too low in fibre-rich plant-based foods. Studies indicate that only a minority of Westerners have a sufficiently speedy transit time and healthy bowel movement.

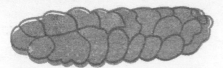

**Type 3** Like a sausage but with cracks in the surface.
Getting better but not ideal.

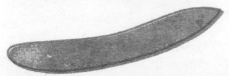

**Type 4** Like a sausage or snake, smooth and soft. This is what stools should look like – at least most of the time – on a healthy fibre-rich diet, indicating a fast transit time. They glide out smoothly and comfortably requiring no conscious effort or straining. Afterwards you are left with such a pleasant feeling of relief that loo visits even feature among life's little pleasures.

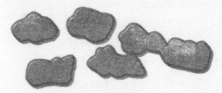

**Type 5** Soft blobs with clear-cut edges. Not all healthy stools will look like Type 4, above. Some, particularly those passed later in the day after the morning bowel movement, can be more broken up without being liquid. Stools of this nature are just as healthy as long as passed effortlessly rather than urgently.

## VIEW FROM THE LOO (CONTINUED)

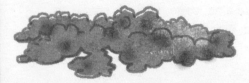

**Type 6** Fluffy pieces with ragged edges, a mushy stool, may indicate you are overstimulating transit time – and a liquid or near-liquid stool certainly would. As with everything else, it is possible to take too much fibre, particularly cereal fibre, and to increase your intake too quickly. It can take a little time to tune your body to a healthy diet if you are used to a fibre-depleted Western diet. Some high-fibre foods upset some people who are specially sensitive to them. Grainy breads might not be well tolerated, for instance. If this problem arises, switch to stoneground or kibbled wholemeal bread instead. And delay introducing the highest-fibre wheat-based cereal for a while.

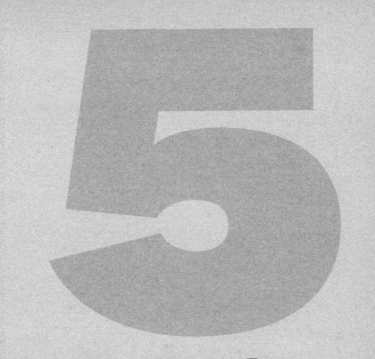

# THE BIG WEIGHT-LOSS BONUS

' The majority of studies show that high intake of NSP (dietary fibre) promotes weight loss.'

THE WORLD HEALTH ORGANIZATION

SO FAR we've focused on health benefits other than loss of surplus weight. But for weight loss alone a fibre-rich diet offers the most effective formula by far for ease and speed.

Calories are all that count when it comes to weight loss. But the source of those calories will largely determine the number you eat and, to some extent, the percentage your body uses. Here are just some of the reasons why those living on high-fibre diets rarely gain weight. And why switching to this eating pattern will painlessly whisk away accumulated surplus:

## You get more food for fewer calories

The foods which can be eaten in the largest quantity for the lowest cost in calories are all plant foods. Nearly all vegetables and fruit are virtually fat free, and many are highly diluted with no-calorie water. Even the more calorie-dense grain-based foods such as most breads and breakfast cereals rate as moderate rather than high in calories.

# More calories are wasted

On a high-fibre diet you will shed fat faster than on any other diet of the same number of calories. This is well-proven scientific fact.

Not all the calories we consume are used for energy or fat storage. There's a natural wastage of about 5 per cent on any diet. On a high-fibre diet this wastage is significantly increased – often more than doubled. This has been demonstrated by many well-controlled scientific studies, not, like some diet claims, on just one outdated, poorly constructed or unsubstantiated study.

By adding more fibre to your diet you are likely to excrete about a hundred more undigested calories a day in faeces, giving a useful boost to weight loss. Within reasonable limits, the more fibre you eat the more calories you excrete. Young men with hearty appetites have been found to excrete more than two hundred extra calories daily on high-fibre diets.

The main component of dietary fibre is calorie-free and we now know that approximately 10 per cent of the starch in carbohydrate foods remains undigested. Fibre encourages good bacteria to grow and that too increases the number of calories lost in faeces.

High-fibre diets really DO offer the proven weight-loss bonus that many mistakenly sought on high-protein diets.

## You feel more satisfied

It's strange, but true, that the longer it takes to chew food the fewer calories you are likely to consume. Studies show this affects not only mental and physical appetite-control systems, but also – more surprisingly – the length of time elapsing before you feel hungry again.

What was it they used to say: a second on the lips, a lifetime on the hips? All too true of those slip-down-in-seconds fatty foods like rich dairy ice-creams, creamy desserts, cheesecake, chocolate, crisps, cream cheese, mayonnaise, buttery and cheesy sauces. Hundreds of calories can slip down the throat in foods like these before they even begin to register on appetite-control mechanisms.

In its report on global obesity, the World Health Organization warns of the 'passive overconsumption' caused by high-fat diets which overwhelm mental and physical satiety signals: 'fat-induced appetite-control signals are thought to be too weak, or too delayed, to prevent the rapid intake of energy (calories) from a fatty meal'.

It takes up to five minutes for food put in the mouth to even start to satisfy the body; up to twenty for it to fill the stomach and send out all the physical signals of sufficiency. Studies have shown that the overweight eat at a considerably faster rate than the slim. Combine fast eating and high-fat diets and you begin to understand the modern phenomenon of sofa-sized people.

Highly refined carbohydrates, such as sugar, white bread and other cereal foods which have been stripped of their fibre, are fast foods too. But when carbohydrates retain their cell-wall material, their fibre, more chewing is

# THE ULTIMATE FIBRE-EATER

The world's greatest fibre-eater is the giant panda – an animal which certainly takes things far too far! The panda eats only bamboo. Only one sixth of what it eats is digested, whole leaves are excreted in its poo, and as a result the panda must munch for fourteen hours a day merely to maintain its weight.

Happily, humans can ensure a high-fibre intake on an attractive and varied diet, but similar principles apply – lots of food can be eaten at low calorie cost and some of the calories will be helpfully excreted to speed weight loss.

involved, significantly extending eating time. Consider how long it would take to chomp your way through four apples, compared to the speed at which you could swig down their juice (basically just the apple stripped of its fibre) and you get an excellent illustration of yet another major weight-loss benefit of high-fibre diets.

## Your 'tum' is full

Dietary fibre is a sponge-like material which absorbs and holds water as it is chewed and passes down the gastro-intestinal tract. This means that fibre-rich foods swell to a greater bulk than other foods, making them more effective in filling the stomach.

Once in the stomach, most of these foods give gastric acids a tough job in fighting their way through cell-wall material. So the stomach not only fills up more but stays full for longer.

## Your blood sugar levels stay steady

Once digested in the intestine, all carbohydrates are absorbed into the bloodstream in the form of sugar to provide essential fuel for body and brain. Some carbohy-drates, mainly those highly processed and stripped of fibre, tend to be absorbed too fast, raising blood sugar levels too quickly. Others, mainly those in nature's packaging which you will be eating on this diet, are absorbed at a slower and more desirable rate for health and weight control.

But here we've reached a hot topical dieting issue – the Glycaemic Index. Read on and be assured that for all but diabetics, who have their own necessarily stricter rules, blood sugar level will be controlled for maximum health and appetite benefits by **F2**.

# THE EASY GUIDE TO GI

THE GLYCAEMIC INDEX is a measure of the extent to which the carbohydrate in different foods raises blood sugar levels. This science-based concept has been subject to some pretty silly misinterpretations in recent years, not least in being used to claim health virtues for unhealthy low-carbohydrate diets. It is, however, of great importance to diabetics and can affect the rest of us too. Some scientists believe that blood sugar raised too high too often can be a factor in causing diabetes and other health problems. In weight control it is one of several factors – not, in my view, the major factor, and certainly not the single factor.

## So what are the facts?

All carbohydrates are converted into blood sugar to provide fuel for body and mind – a normal, healthy and necessary process. Very necessary, for instance, if you'd prefer your brain to carry on functioning. Carbohydrate is the only fuel the brain can use, and the brain actually uses more calories than it takes to keep the whole of the rest of the body ticking over.

Medical literature shows that, starved of carbohydrate for too long, the brain functions less efficiently in many ways. Mental judgement is impaired. When blood sugar levels fall below a certain threshold dizziness, nausea, lack of coordination, trembling and much more serious consequences can result. Athletes, if they allow themselves to use up all their carbohydrate reserves, simply collapse.

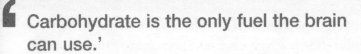

# 'Carbohydrate is the only fuel the brain can use.'

Recent research reveals that different carbohydrate foods have differing effects on blood sugar levels. Some, the high-GI carbs, are speedily digested in the intestine and absorbed into the blood, raising the sugar levels very high, very fast. Others, the low-GI carbs, are digested and absorbed more gradually, raising blood sugar levels more slowly and to a lesser extent.

The body has a control mechanism to keep blood sugar levels on an even keel. When blood sugar increases after we eat carbohydrate the pancreas secretes insulin, a hormone which helps the sugar move out of the blood into other bodily tissues, causing sugar levels in the blood to fall. After a meal which raises blood sugar very high, very fast, the pancreas has to produce a large quantity of insulin. This can lead to blood sugar decreasing to even lower levels than before the meal. When blood sugar is low we tend to feel hungry.

What we need is a slow, steady increase in blood sugar levels, followed by a slow decrease, not dipping too low.

So many factors are involved in stimulating us to eat – the sight or smell of a particular food, the mood we're in, sheer habit, a row, that missed train, a bad day – as well as those physical appetite-control factors already discussed, that to attach undue importance to this one single factor can lead to some pretty silly conclusions. Even dangerous conclusions such as: 'Since only carbohydrate foods raise blood sugar levels the answer is to cut out all carbohydrate foods'!

Top world GI expert Professor Jennie Brand-Miller of the University of Sydney, where much of the GI research has been pioneered, is not in favour of low-carb diets for either weight loss or health. She believes starchy foods to be among the best you can eat to fill you up, stave off hunger pangs and help you lose weight. In *The New Glucose Revolution* (published in the UK by Hodder Mobius), she makes it clear that the GI was never meant to be the sole determinant of which foods are good for us – for example, crisps have a lower GI than baked potatoes and many biscuits a lower GI than bread: 'In these instances a lower GI doesn't mean an automatically better choice from a nutritional standpoint. Saturated fat in these foods will have adverse effects on coronary health far greater than the benefit of lower glucose levels.'

The words 'babies' and 'bathwater' come to mind when one considers the crazy concept of throwing out the foods which lower cholesterol and stimulate anti-cancer bacterial action in favour of fatty foods which do just the opposite.

Sugar in the blood is necessary – indeed, essential. Frequently raising its levels to sudden peaks is all that needs to be avoided. This problem only tends to arise on modern Western diets because so much food has been overprocessed, removing almost all of the fibre.

The fibre factor is by far the most important in ensuring a healthily low GI diet. You are extremely unlikely to experience high glycaemic peaks on a high-fibre diet.

But what makes specific foods desirably low or undesirably high on the GI index is a complex business also depending, to a lesser extent, on a variety of additional factors. In fact a multiplicity of factors, such as starch

‘ **The fibre factor is by far the most important in ensuring a healthily low GI diet.'**

gelatinization, high amylose to amylopectin ratio . . . don't ask! That is why all foods have to be laboriously tested individually to determine their GI. And why many foods have not yet been tested.

Happily, you are unlikely to run into blood-sugar problems when you follow the **F2** fibre-rich formula. But on the following pages you will find some 'belt and braces' tips to ensure your blood sugar is kept on an even keel for health and appetite control.

# ALL YOU REALLY NEED TO KNOW (THANK HEAVENS!) ABOUT THE GLYCAEMIC INDEX

No need to agonize about the GI values of all the foods you eat. It's the GI of whole meals that determines their impact on speed of blood-sugar release. Unless you suffer from diabetes, in which case you will be familiar with your own special dietary rules, the **F2** formula keeps your blood-sugar levels on an even keel for health and appetite control because of its high fibre content and the following factors:

➤ **Minimally ground grains:** the less finely ground wholemeal breads recommended on **F2** helpfully slow the release of sugar into the bloodstream as well as speeding transit time in the colon.

## GLYCAEMIC INDEX (CONTINUED)

➤ **Loads of legumes:** beans, lentils, chickpeas and peas are richly represented in **F2**'s stand-by salads and soups, the mainstay of your menus. These have an exceptionally low GI and effectively lower the GI of meals.

➤ **Lots of fruit:** those fruits recommended on page 91 for their high fibre content are all low-GI fruits. People who eat three or four servings of fruit daily, as you will on **F2**, have been found to have the lowest overall GI and the best blood-sugar control.

➤ **Plenty of pasta:** you are not only allowed to but encouraged to eat wholewheat pasta meals on **F2**, and all pasta has a low GI.

## GI-LOWERING TIPS

**1** **Use acidic fruits to further lower the GI of meals.** Both their fibre and acids are thought to be responsible for their significant effect in slowing down stomach emptying. The more acidic the fruit the lower its GI. Hence half a grapefruit, which is part of your **F2** breakfast, can make a marked difference to the speed of sugar absorption from the meal.

All citrus fruits have a low GI – as have fruits grown in temperate climes, apples, pears, plums, strawberries and other berries. Tropical fruits such mango and pineapple have an intermediate GI. Bananas, as eaten while still a little green on **F2**, have a lower GI than the riper fruit.

**2** **Lash on the lemon juice.** This enhances the flavour of fish dishes and soups, providing a particularly easy way to slow gastric emptying and lower the GI of meals. Add a little lemon juice to the water you drink with your meal, or try a slice of lemon rather than milk in your tea.

**3** **Use vinegar, which has the same beneficial acidic impact.** A vinaigrette dressing on an **F2** side-salad helps control the blood-sugar response to a whole meal.

**4** **Partner your potatoes with low GI legumes – peas, beans or chickpeas.** This way you don't have to sacrifice the delicious, nutritious and fibre-rich baked potato, just because it happens to be one of the very few high GI veg.

**5** **Don't even worry about GI when eating other veg.** Legumes are low GI. Carrots, sweet potatoes and sweetcorn are moderately low. And leafy vegetables and low-calorie ones like mushrooms, onions and peppers have no measurable effect on blood sugar.

# 7

# CAN YOU GET SLIM WITHOUT EXERCISE?

UNDENIABLE FACT: losing weight depends on eating fewer calories (which are units of energy) than your body uses in moving around and keeping itself functioning. This forces it to draw on its own fat stores for extra fuel. In theory, therefore, there are two ways of losing weight.

➤ One is to eat fewer calories.

➤ The other is to increase energy output by exercising more so that you burn up more calories.

REALISTIC FACT: it is perfectly possible to lose weight by sufficiently reducing calorie intake even if you don't take more exercise. By following the **F2** formula alone you can shed surplus weight.

In contrast, it is exceedingly difficult to shed any significant amount of surplus weight by exercise alone if you don't also adjust your diet. This would require a very great deal of time, effort, persistence and patience.

Cutting down on the calories you eat is far more effective.

When I tell you that you'd have to walk about 50 miles at a pretty brisk pace in order to shed a pound you'll see why the 'exercise-alone' solution isn't a realistic answer for most people's weight problems. In terms of calorie-burning, most forms of exercise produce similarly modest results.

If exercise is part and parcel of your life – if you are doing heavy manual work and expending considerable energy throughout your working day, for instance – this will certainly make a significant difference to your weight. But if exercise is an 'add on', something you decide to do for a couple of hours a couple of times a week, or for twenty minutes a day, in order to solve your weight problem, you are unlikely to be a happy bunny when you step on the scales.

Of course, 'add-on' exercise of the right type taken to sufficient lengths could achieve significant weight loss. Taking up regular long-distance running and training for the London marathon would do it. Not a surplus ounce on our Paula! But are you a marathon-make of man or woman?

Most people who decide to tackle their weight problems want to do so in weeks or months, not years. And why not? In most cases the exercise-alone solution can only get you to your target by the very slow track.

Public bodies, anxious to avoid offending the food industry, sometimes focus on exercise as the main answer to obesity. What's to upset anyone in advising: 'Take more exercise'? Never underestimate the politics of food.

Yet, despite all this, I strongly recommend you work out ways to get more active as you start F2, for all the following reasons:

# Health

Exercise improves blood circulation and strengthens the heart. Lack of it is also thought to be the major cause of osteoporosis. Regular weight-bearing exercise is the best thing you can do for your bones. This needn't involve actually lifting weights – lifting or moving the weight of your own body, as in walking, jogging, playing sport or doing press-ups, for example, will do it.

# Metabolism

Although exercise alone is rarely enough to solve a weight problem, it can give a rewarding little speed boost to weight loss as you follow **F2**.

Exercise burns extra calories both while you do it and after you stop. The boost it gives to metabolic rate – the rate at which your body burns up calories – lasts for up to two hours afterwards. A really brisk walk, a jog, skipping, a game of tennis, anything that makes you 'glow' will have this dual impact – not enough to make you slim, but enough to speed dieting weight loss.

The best calorie-burning exercises are those which involve moving your whole body from place to place, the faster the better. Better still, moving it against gravity. A quick jog up Mount Everest would certainly do the trick – even if you stuffed your rucksack with Mars bars and cheese. I once knew a mountaineer who used to shed about two stone on his way up Himalayan peaks. In more realistic terms, Tai Chi and yoga (other than Ashtanga 'power yoga'), while offering other excellent benefits, aren't significant calorie burners. However, any type of exercise session in which you carry your body weight, even if it's up and down a step in the gym, and which leaves you damp, pink and in need of a shower, is.

' A quick jog up Mount Everest would certainly do the trick – even if you stuffed your rucksack with Mars bars and cheese.'

## Mood

Exercise is a scientifically proven antidote to the depression which so often leads to comfort eating or diet-breaking. During a difficult period in my younger years I discovered this for myself, and went on to research the scientific reasons. When you exercise with any vigour, even with a brisk walk, you manufacture your own powerful mood-lifting chemicals. You give yourself a chemical kick to cure the blues. And the impact lasts for some time afterwards. Please try it, and surprise yourself by its effect, as I did, next time you are in a low mood.

Boredom is an equally dangerous mood for dieters. Signing up for regular exercise sessions, packing your spare time with positive mood-enhancing activities, puts you in the right frame of mind to keep to your diet.

## Looks

No need to go for a Madonna-like muscle-bulge (call me old-fashioned, but I'm not keen on that, are you?), but a firm, well-exercised slim figure looks even better than a slim figure.

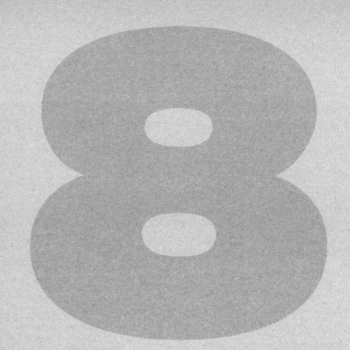

# THE KNOTTY ISSUE OF STAYING SLIM

I DON'T KNOW ABOUT YOU, but that phrase 'this is a diet you can follow for the rest of your life' somehow fills me with profound depression. Let's consider how F2 can help you keep slim once you've reached your target weight, without sending you rushing for the Prozac.

First, the good news: you can consume significantly more calories when just aiming to control your weight than when you are actually working at shedding weight. The latter requires that you eat fewer calories than your body needs, while the former means eating just enough to supply your body's requirements. It's hard to quantify the difference precisely, so much depends on height and gender, but it would amount to several hundred calories daily. If you have lost several stone your body will have temporarily adjusted, to some degree, to famine conditions, so at first you must eat less food to avoid weight gain than you will be able to eat later.

In place of the word 'calories' think in terms of the word 'fat', because we're all aware by now, I trust, that the fat in the diet is by far the main source of all those surplus calories. So to stay slim you will still have to control fat intake – but not to the same strict degree.

But here's a realistic question that I want you to ask yourself and answer honestly: Do you believe that, having shed all your surplus on F2, you will stay at the same target weight for the rest of your life? No, I don't either. Those prone to weight gain are also prone to fluctuate by at least a few pounds. There are holidays, bad days, bad weeks ... Too many diets are written by men who have little understanding of the emotional factors that can lead women to overeat. The psychological key to post-diet weight control is to resolutely set a maximum weight over which **you will not allow yourself to go**. Stand like Horatio on that spot. I'd advise seven pounds of surplus weight as the absolute maximum – three or four pounds would be much better. Get back on F2's ten fat units a day as soon as you reach that maximum, or, better still, follow the F2 Fast Track Tactics on page 100.

However, having shed your surplus weight on F2's healthy and highly effective formula, you will have learned and practised much that will be of immense value in helping you to stay slim in the future. Here are just some of the factors that will work to your advantage:

## No more 'accidental calories'

Two categories of foods lie behind weight problems:

➤ Foods you simply didn't realize were so fattening.

➤ Foods you know to be fattening but find hard to resist.

Consumption of the former has been much increased in the backwash of the late, unlamented low-carb craze. You still see people 'virtuously' waving away bread and potatoes then piling into the much higher calorie saturated-fat packed cheese. Mistakes like that, which they've been encouraged to make, make me really hate that diet (in case you hadn't noticed!).

**F2**'s Fat and Calorie Controller sorts out such confusion once and for all. I don't believe you'll ever again lash on the oil in the mistaken belief that because it's 'healthy oil' it won't impact on your weight, or consider a mayonnaise-rich supermarket coleslaw a harmless addition to a meal – 'it's only salad' – or down a couple of mini Scotch eggs as a little 'can't add up to much' snack.

In relation to those foods you always knew to be fattening, the quantity-control tactics recommended in **F2**'s Fat and Calorie Controller will help a lot. When I experience an occasional chocolate craving I call in at Thornton's and get them to count out just five of my favourite chocs (don't ask 'Why five?' – that just seems to do it for me).

## New 'balance' in your way of eating

When people tell me of health problems clearly related to what they eat and I tentatively mutter something about diet, they always, *always* insist, 'Oh, but I follow a healthy balanced diet already.'

They don't. They think they do. The truth is that the typical British diet has moved so far away from healthy balance in the last half-century that most people don't even know what a healthy balanced diet is. That's why I long to shoot those experts who parrot the pointless phrase 'as long as you follow a healthy balanced diet'. Quelle cop-out!

**F2**, with its major emphasis on fibre-rich plant foods and a low proportion of animal products, at least shows you what a healthy balanced diet really means and allows you to start to experience the benefits.

' The truth is that the typical British diet has moved so far away from healthy balance in the last half-century that most people don't even know what a healthy balanced diet is.'

The bad news is that deeply instilled eating habits don't change overnight, nor even in the weeks or months it might take to solve a weight problem.

The good news is that, with persistence, they do change, steadily, gradually and increasingly, until good eating habits actually become effortless preferences. The more vegetables you eat with a meal the more you start to like vegetables. The wholemeal bread you get used to eating becomes the bread you like. And, after you've reduced fatty foods for a time, although this may take months, you begin to find them too greasy and naturally gravitate to lower-fat options.

Decades of observation have convinced me that what I call 'the throw-up threshold' can, in time, adjust. Let me explain:

When so-called 'naturally thin' people say, 'I honestly couldn't eat another mouthful,' in most cases they really mean it. The prospect of eating more, particularly when the food is rich (fatty!), is positively nauseating to them.

This happened to me the other day when I greedily accepted (I put it down to the wine!) 'a little bit of each' of two delectable desserts at a dinner party. Much as I hated the thought of offending my hostess, appetite control mechanisms, acquired in my case over the years, forced me to a reluctant and embarrassed full stop half way through the dish.

Observe, in contrast, as I was taught to do by a leading expert in eating behaviour, very fat people eating meals. Clearly they have a very high 'throw-up threshold' – if any at all. They are able to eat a quantity of rich, fatty food that would make the rest of us physically sick. Physical and psychological stop mechanisms have collapsed completely.

For the vast majority with more moderate weight problems it is more a matter of the 'throw-up-threshold' having been slightly raised by a lifetime of eating a typical fatty Western diet. With a little persistence it can be lowered. And then weight control – I promise – really does become effortless.

But we're running ahead of ourselves. First we've got your weight problem to solve. Let's get started, shall we?

# PART

# 2

# HOW TO FOLLOW F2

# THE SUPER-HEALTHY FORMULA FOR FAST WEIGHT LOSS

FOLLOW THESE RULES to lose weight fast and revitalize your health. **F2** boosts the quantity of fibre you eat from all three vital sources – fruit, vegetables and grains – packing meals with powerful protective nutrients as it cuts harmful fatty calories. For most people **F2**'s healthy 40 grams of fibre daily will double present fibre intake. You'll feel the difference as your good bacteria flourish. You'll see the difference as surplus pounds melt away.

**F2** changes the balance of your diet, making plant-based foods the mainstay. 'Five portions of fruit and veg a day'? This UK recommendation is merely a minimum goal designed to move diets in the right direction. Recent research indicates that it takes much more, plus a significant quantity of wholegrain foods, to gain maximum health benefit. The **F2** formula will show you what healthy eating *really* means. And just how good it makes you feel.

First we've listed the rules in brief, but please read the more detailed explanations that follow.

# THE DIET RULES

**1** **Breakfast** on half a grapefruit, a bowl of one of the recommended cereals, and a 'just ripe' greenish banana.

**2** Have a low-fat probiotic drink or yogurt each day.

**3** Pre-prepare **F2** Soups and Salads (pages 104–19). Eat them as meals, or with meals, frequently – include at least one or two servings in your menu each day.

**4** Pile into large quantities of vegetables and pulses including at least two of the **F2** Star Bioactive Veg and Pulses, listed on page 85, daily.

**5** Boost your fruit by eating at least two of the **F2** Star Bioactive Fruits (page 90) daily, in addition to your breakfast banana and grapefruit.

**6** Eat fibre-rich wholemeal bread: two slices daily.

**7** Feel free to enjoy these grain-based foods: wholewheat pasta, brown basmati rice, couscous, noodles, barley and bulgur wheat.

**8** **Ration fat-containing foods**, listed in the **F2** Fat and Calorie Controller chart on pages 128–58, to a maximum of 10 units daily.

**9** **Choose fish in preference to meat**, or follow a vegetarian menu. Limit any red or processed meat to a maximum of two portions a week in total and select only organic or free-range animal products.

**10** **Drink** water, teas and most low-calorie drinks freely and coffee in moderation. See full details about drinks on page 94.

**Take a glance at our sample menus (pages 184–92) to see just how easy F2 eating will be – then read the 'how to' details on the following pages.**

## Before you begin

Follow these vital preparation tactics:

## Cook F2 soups

Spend a weekend morning or evening cooking and freezing large quantities of at least two of the soups on pages 104 –11. Never let supplies run out. These soups are a vital part of the **F2** formula to:

● Boost your daily intake of the fibre that speeds weight loss and feeds good bacteria.

● Lower the GI level of meals at which they are eaten, and even the meals which follow.

● Provide you with an always-available low-calorie snack or light meal. Diet disaster is a done deal if you find yourself with only fattening food in the house.

## Prepare **F2** several-day salads

Make at least two fibre-rich salads from pages 112–19 and store under cling-film in the fridge for all the same reasons. They stay fresh for several days, so you can make several servings in one session. Pay special attention to the way you dress your salads. You'll find all the info you need on pages 120–1.

## More cooking chores?

Apart from cooking lots of veg, that's all of the 'essential' cooking. After that you can put together menus as time-taking or time-saving as you wish. The more you cook, storing meals in the fridge and freezer, the easier and healthier your diet will be. But by far the most important factor for weight loss and health is the change in balance from high-fat to high-fibre plant-based meals. For busy people, **F2** allows shortcuts to make this switch possible.

# Probiotic drinks and yogurts

A wide selection of milk drinks and yogurts claiming various bacterial benefits are now available. Choose those labelled low fat, light or fat free. The word 'probiotic' on the label means they should contain live bacteria capable of surviving the journey through your digestive system to supplement the good bacteria in your gut.

**Suitable low-fat probiotic drinks and yogurts:**

● Yakult Light probiotic drink

● Actimel Yogurt probiotic drink (.01% fat)

● Muller Vitality low-fat probiotic yogurt or drink

# The F2 fast-forward breakfast

**Wheat fibre is the outstanding 'fast-forward' fibre,** the most effective, by far, in speeding waste matter through the gut. It has consistently been shown to be the most protective against cancer. Most corn-based cereals don't contain sufficient fibre to speed transit time, and oat fibre has little impact in this respect. Kellogg's All-Bran Original, the cereal which contains the most wheat fibre, is also one of the lowest-GI cereals.

'Neat' bran of any nature, with its lightness and sawdust taste and texture, is hard to eat in quantity. You need to spoon in a surprisingly large volume to get much benefit.

Fibre-rich wheat-based breakfast cereals make it easier to eat an effective quantity.

However, it's wise to increase fibre intake gradually, particularly that from grains, so we suggest you breakfast on fibre-rich bran flakes when you start eating the **F2** way. Then gradually mix in a little of the very high fibre All-Bran Original, stepping up the quantity to as much as suits.

## **F2** bioactive cereals

● Kellogg's All-Bran Original – 27% fibre, 11g in an average 40g serving.

● Kellogg's All-Bran Bran Flakes – 15% fibre, 4.5g in an average 30g serving.

● Kellogg's All-Bran Sultana Bran – 13% fibre, 5.2g in an average 40g serving.

## Breakfast reminders

● Start with half a grapefruit, for its GI-lowering impact and Vitamin C. Pink grapefruit are sweeter and help you resist sugar.

● Slice your greenish banana into your cereal and sweeten with a small spoon of sultanas if you wish. Add soya or skimmed milk – or your probiotic milk drink.

## Breakfast alternative

If you long for toast, breakfast once a week on two slices of wholemeal toast in addition to your daily allowance (a Sunday-morning treat?). Help yourself in moderation to honey, jam or marmalade but subtract fat units for any fat spreads used.

## Wheat allergies

Only a very small minority of people are genuinely allergic to wheat, but, of late, unqualified practitioners have encouraged many to think that they are. This has not been good news in such a constipated nation. Rye is also effective in speeding transit time and those who can tolerate it could breakfast on rye toast – doubling their total daily bread allowance. Many health-food shops sell fibre-rich rye bread.

Those restricted to oats should opt for an unrefined muesli with large oat flakes and add plenty of chopped prunes, figs and dates.

# Star bioactive veg and pulses

**Aim to eat approximately 15 grams of fibre from vegetables and pulses as a daily average.** We've listed the fibre quantity in the richest sources on pages 88 and 89. Your daily quantity of fibre can fluctuate to a degree – a little more on some days, a little less on others. Make vegetables and pulses the mainstay of main meals, not just a side issue, and be sure to include the following:

**Pulses:** beans, peas and lentils. High in fibre, rich in resistant starch, these rate very high among the best protective plant foods. Recent research reveals eating more of them to be the best thing you can do for the whole of your body, not just your gut. That's why the latest (2005) US government dietary guidelines recommend that pulses should be consumed several times a week. As well as feeding good bacteria they significantly lower bad cholesterol in the blood, help prevent blood sugar levels rising too high and supply particularly valuable nutrients such as iron and B vitamins. We've put plenty into **F2**'s Essential Soups and Salads to make it easy to include a daily portion in your menus.

There are many varieties of beans and all are rich in fibre content. Estimate a minimum of 5.5g fibre for any variety of bean (out of the pod) not listed in the chart that follows. Dried beans, when they have been soaked and cooked, will supply a similar quantity of fibre to the same weight of canned beans.

**Onions and their relatives,** shallots and leeks, are rising bioactive stars. Recent studies reveal that your ultra-good bifidobacteria flourish on the oligosaccharides they supply.

**Bright-red, orange and dark-green veg** are rich sources of cancer-preventive antioxidants and minerals.

**All vegetables,** with the exception of fat-rich avocados, should be eaten in generous quantities on **F2**. Aim to at least double your usual quantity, serve two or three with a meal. Include two of the highest-fibre varieties, featured on pages 88 and 89, daily – most are included in **F2** Salads and Soups, making this easy.

When serving baked potatoes always combine this high-GI veg with low-GI foods (see Baked Potato Easy Meals, page 174). It's the GI of the whole meal that counts in keeping blood sugar levels steady.

# FAT ALERT:

**Adding fat to veg makes calories soar. Some vegetables, such as aubergine, and mushrooms, soak it up insatiably during cooking, as do potatoes cooked in fat to make crisps or chips.**

● Count any oil or fat used in cooking or serving vegetables as part of the ten units allowed daily on the Fat and Calorie Controller.

● Avoid using fat when cooking veg if possible.

● Invest in a new non-stick frying pan if yours has seen better days; even a single teaspoon of oil goes a long way in the right pan.

● Equip yourself with a special brush or oil drizzler to baste veg with only the tiniest quantity of oil when grilling or baking.

● Consider investing in a steamer in which several veg can be cooked fat-free at the same time – a great aid for weight control and health.

# VEGETABLE

Approx grams
fibre in portion

### Lentils:
40g/1½oz raw-weight portion — **9**

### Peas:
generous 150g/5oz portion — **8**

### Pinto beans:
small 215g can — **8**

### Baked beans in tomato sauce:
200g can — **8**

### Red kidney beans:
half a 410g can — **8**

### Cannellini beans:
half a 410g can — **7**

### Baked potato:
200g/7oz raw weight eaten with skin* — **7**

### Butter beans:
half a 410g can — **6**

### Mixed beans:
half a 410g can* — **5.5**

### Parsnips:
175g/6oz raw weight — **5.5**

### Chickpeas:
half a 410g can — **5**

### Sweet potato:
175g/6oz raw weight — **5**

| | Approx grams fibre in portion |
|---|---|
| **Brussels sprouts:** 200g/7oz raw weight | 5 |
| **Mushy peas:** half a 300g can | 5 |
| **Carrots:** two medium-sized, 175g/6oz raw weight in total | 5 |
| **Sweetcorn kernels:** small 200g can | 4 |
| **Sugarsnap peas:** 115g/4oz raw weight | 3 |
| **Mangetout:** 100g/3½oz raw weight | 3 |
| **Broccoli:** 115g/4oz raw weight | 3 |
| **Spinach:** 100g/3½oz raw weight | 2.5 |
| **Green runner beans:** 100g/3½oz raw weight | 2.5 |
| **Cabbage:** 100g/3½oz raw weight | 2 |
| **Leeks:** 150g/5oz raw weight | 1.5 |

# Star bioactive fruits

**Aim to eat approximately 10 grams of fruit fibre daily.** Again this can fluctuate a little from day to day. Fruit fibre feeds good bacteria in the gut, helps lower bad cholesterol in the blood, and offers a multitude of health benefits. Many fruits, citrus fruit and berries in particular, have a high content of the protective antioxidant Vitamin C. People who eat three or four servings of fruit daily have also been found to have the lowest overall GI and best blood sugar control.

**Start breakfast with half a grapefruit.** Calorie content is very low, Vitamin C content is very high, and acidic fruits like this are particularly helpful in lowering the GI of a meal. Go very easy on any added sugar. Part-sugar sweetening products can help and you will find that pink grapefruit doesn't need sweetening.

Half a grapefruit supplies approx 1.5 grams fibre.

**Eat at least one medium-sized greenish banana each day.** This is one of the best sources of resistant starch, which has the greatest impact in stimulating good bacteria to produce butyrate, a powerful anti-cancer agent. To achieve this bio-benefit a banana must be only just ripe, with skin still a little green. On full ripening, the resistant starch converts to sugar. Buy the greenest bananas you can find, just a few at a time.

A medium-sized banana supplies approx 3 grams fibre.

**In addition eat approximately 5–6 grams of fibre from fibre-rich, low-GI fruits each day.** They are listed on the chart in descending order of fibre content supplied by an average-sized fruit or serving – superfruits at the top.

| FRUIT | Approx grams fibre |
|---|---|
| **Blackberries or raspberries** (bowlful) | 6 |
| **Pear** | 5 |
| **Orange** | 5 |
| **Apple** | 3 |
| **Strawberries** (bowlful) | 2.5 |
| **Cherries** (average portion) | 2.5 |
| **Nectarine** | 2.5 |
| **Kiwi fruit** | 2.5 |
| **Blueberries** (half a 150g pack) | 2 |
| **Small bunch of grapes** | 1.5 |
| **Peach** | 1.5 |
| **Clementine, mandarin or satsuma** | 1.5 |
| **Plum** | 1 |

**Cautionary note about dried fruits (sultanas, currants, raisins, etc.)** Eat only in small quantities as part of a meal, to sweeten your breakfast cereal or as an ingredient in a salad, for instance. You risk packing down too many calories if you snack on dried fruit 'neat'.

**Canned fruit** Fresh fruit offers greater nutritional advantage, but if you eat canned fruit occasionally choose varieties canned in fruit juice rather than higher-calorie syrup.

# The **F2** good grains

Aim to eat approximately 15 grams cereal fibre (including that in your breakfast cereal) daily. Cereal-based foods which supply dietary fibre, resistant starch and a variety of vitamins and minerals are good foods for your health-protective bacteria and great foods for dieting. Eat these 'complex carbohydrates' on **F2** in preference to refined carbs, like white flour and sugar.

## Best **F2** bread

Choose wholemeal bread and enjoy up to 115g/4oz – two slices of a large loaf – each day. This will contribute approximately 6 grams of fibre. No need to eat your full quota on days when it may not fit into your chosen menu and when meals include other grain-based foods such as wholewheat pasta.

Transit time and other health benefits are reduced and GI raised when grains are too finely ground. Wholemeal breads labelled 'kibbled' or 'stoneground' are among the less finely ground. If you are breakfasting on the recommended wheat-based cereals, you can opt for a different type of grain for your bread if you wish.

**Start on 'kibbled' or 'stoneground' wholemeal breads. Try visibly grainy breads when you have become accustomed to a high fibre diet.**

To locate visibly grainy breads check out health-food stores, where local makes are sometimes available, and specialist-bread sections in supermarkets, where you will usually find the following:

- German-style rye bread such as Bolletje (very grainy, mainly rye but also contains some wheat bran)

- Burgen Soya and Linseed Loaf

- Vogel Sunflower and Barley or Soya and Linseed Bread

- Vogel Original Mixed Grain Brown Bread

**Wholemeal pitta bread:** a good alternative choice for fibre. A wholemeal pitta weighs approx 50g/2oz. Include it in your daily bread ration if you wish.

# CAUTION:

Some people are sensitive to ingredients in some grainy breads. If visiting the bathroom too often, revert to a stoneground or kibbled wholemeal.

## Pasta

Pasta is a superfood on many scores. Brown pasta is a very rich source of fibre. Cold pasta is a particularly valuable source of the resistant starch which stimulates good bacteria to produce cancer-preventing butyrate. And all pasta, even white pasta, has a low GI and a reasonably low calorie content. Choose brown wholewheat pasta and eat it freely with low-fat sauces from our recipes or fat-counted ready-mades.

## Rice

Choose brown basmati. Basmati has the lowest GI of all rice and brown rice has a higher fibre content than white rice.

## Bulgar wheat, couscous

Useful fat-free staples for dieting meals. Enjoy freely.

## Barley

High fibre, low GI – add it freely to soups and stews.

# What (and what not) to drink

Every calorie you drink is a costly calorie. It does nothing to satisfy hunger and is surplus to the calories you eat. Don't 'waste' calories on sugary drinks, which are often surprisingly high in calories, when so many virtually calorie-free drinks are available.

## Alcohol

Try to avoid drinking alcohol while shedding weight. It is very high in calories. But if, for you, it's a choice between having one glass of wine in the evening and dieting, as opposed to not dieting at all, opt for the former and compensate for the extra calories by following Fast Track **F2** Slimming Tactics on pages 100–1. Restrict your 'glass' of wine to a very modest 140ml/5fl oz. And if you find that one little glass leads to another little glass – as it so often does – bite the bullet and cut alcohol out completely until you're slim.

## Water

Drink as much as you wish. You need at least two litres of fluids a day in total, but fruit and vegetables contribute to fluid intake.

## 'Low calorie' drinks

No limits here, but go easy on the low-calorie colas, choosing flavoured mineral waters instead.

## Fruit juice

Banned – but only while you are shedding weight. Although a rich source of nutrients, juice can also be a rich source of calories. It's all too easy to down the juice of four or more fruits in one drink. When you eat whole fruit it impacts on your appetite. When you only drink the juice it doesn't. But there's one exception here . . .

## Lemon juice

Use as much as you can. Squeeze it on fish, stir it into soups. It supplies too few calories to count, a very high level of health-protecting Vitamin C and, along with other acidic fruit, has a major effect in lowering the GI of meals.

## Coffee

Enjoy in moderation. Old scientific studies giving coffee a particularly bad name were based on non-filtered coffee. Filtered or instant coffee later emerged as much safer bets. But there are still some health concerns which indicate that moderation is best. Sugar? Just the very occasional teaspoon in the very occasional cup wouldn't stop your weight loss, but generally it's best to use a low-calorie sweetener.

# Tea

Feel free to enjoy today's bewildering array, whether you sip Lapsang Souchong from a delicate china teacup or gulp 'workman's' from a big chipped mug. Followers of fashion can indulge in the full range of herbal teas – camomile, ginseng, peppermint, oatstraw (oatstraw?), dandelion and the like. Regular tea drinkers would benefit from drinking tea with a slice of GI-lowering lemon rather than milk. Sugar? Follow the advice given for coffee.

## Milk and alternatives

Skimmed organic dairy milk or unsweetened soya milk are the recommended **F2** choices. Subtract units from your daily ten for the type and quantity you use. Although soya milk contains a little fat it lacks the same high proportion of unhealthy saturated fat present in dairy products. Many studies have shown that soya has an impressive ability to reduce blood cholesterol and some indicate that it protects against breast and prostate cancers. Soya milks labelled 'with calcium' contain as much calcium as dairy milk.

# Why **F2** limits meat

**F2** limits red and processed meat to no more than two small helpings, if any, a week, even if the meat is lean and low in fat. Many scientific studies,* including major recent studies which would be very hard to argue with, have linked high intake of these meats with increased cancer risk. The term 'processed meats' refers to ham, bacon, sausages, luncheon meat, salami, and most delicatessen meats.

Recent research reveals that after meat has been eaten, residues in the large intestine stimulate bacteria to produce carcinogens – substances implicated in causing cancer. On high-meat diets the levels of these dangerous compounds in the colon have been found to be similar to those produced in the lungs by tobacco smoke after smoking.

By replacing meat with fish you also opt for the more beneficial fats.

Vegetarians can cut out both meat and fish and rely on plant-based sources to provide all the nutrients they need. Foods like beans are packed with protein. Generally fitter and slimmer than omnivores, vegetarians tend only to gain weight if they include overgenerous quantities of cheese in their diets – a tendency which is now being discouraged by leading vegetarian organizations.

> \* An analysis of more than one hundred scientific population studies on meat consumption by the International Agency for Research on Cancer concluded: 'The quantitative summary of the published literature suggests that high intake of red meat and processed meat are associated with increased risk of colorectal cancer.'

# How **F2** deals
# with sugar cravings

**F2** rations the many foods which combine fat with sugar – the main source of sugar-related calorie overdoses. You'll find tactics to help you limit these foods in the Fat and Calorie Controller, plus figures which allow you to include them in moderate quantities on days (for many women, those prior to the monthly period) when cravings may become particularly strong. On pages 216–19 we suggest the healthiest way to deal with these cravings – desserts which add extra sweetness to fruit, but which are low in fatty calories and are genuinely easy to make.

**F2** takes a tougher attitude to sugary drinks. Why squander calories on these when so many low-calorie alternatives are available? But sugar can be enjoyed freely in the form of fruit and a little is allowable in other fat-free foods.

A taste of sweetness in many dishes – dried fruit with cereals and salads, sweet chilli sauces – makes **F2** a particularly woman-friendly formula. Allow yourself a taste of honey if you wish. It has been a natural part of the human diet since hunter-gatherer days. Or jam or marmalade, if that's what you prefer. But go easy on quantity. While sugar supplies only half the calories of fat, it is far from being low-calorie.

Few, in our experience, are tempted to binge on sugar in the form of fat-free foods. But if you happen to be a serial sweet-sucker, a sugar-lump cruncher, a dried-fruit nibbler or are drawn like a wasp to the jam, remember that any more than a little can slow or stop weight loss. Sugar

'If you happen to be a serial sweet-sucker or dried-fruit nibbler, remember that more than a little can slow or stop weight loss.'

calories in fruit are highly diluted by water and fibre. In manufactured foods they can be a much more concentrated and significant source of calories.

## And finally...

Pickles, relishes, chilli sauce, ketchup, tomato salsa, etc.: feel free to add that splash of flavour that gives a kick to a dish. Only the fatty ones, such as mayonnaise, need to be rationed by the Fat and Calorie Controller.

## FAST-TRACK F2 SLIMMING TACTICS

**F2**, with its fibre-powered slimming advantage, will ensure an encouragingly speedy weight loss for almost all those with surplus pounds to shed. However, even stricter calorie controls may be helpful in the special circumstances listed over the page.

➤ **You are struggling to polish off the last few pounds** after a prolonged period of dieting (the body may have adjusted to lower calorie intake).

➤ **You are female and small in stature;** the bigger the person the greater the calorie requirement, and men burn up more calories than women.

➤ **You are only a few pounds overweight** and seeking a speedy way to solve a small surplus-weight problem in just two or three weeks.

The following fast-track tactics could be used in these circumstances, or if you have opted to allow yourself a daily glass of wine:

**1** **Lunch on only a bowlful of F2 Soup and a piece of fruit.** The bowl can be as big as you like.

**2** **Restrict fat units to seven a day in total.**

**3** **Ensure that the majority of fat units are spent on foods containing healthy fats.** See Fats – the Facts on page 122 for details.

**4** **Eat fruit freely, but avoid other sweet foods as much as you can.**

# 10

## THE F2 ESSENTIAL SOUPS AND SALADS

READY, STEADY . . . but don't even think of starting until you've made some of these!

These stand-by soups and salads are an essential part of the F2 formula. They:

➤ Boost your intake of resistant starch and dietary fibre to speed weight loss and make your good bacteria flourish.

➤ Pack your diet with 'pulse-power' to lower bad cholesterol and benefit your whole body.

➤ Up your intake of those foods which feed ultra-good bifidobacteria.

➤ Lower the GI of meals to keep blood sugar levels on an even keel.

➤ Provide you with a constant supply of low-fat, low-calorie light meals and snacks.

➤ Make a world of difference to the ease with which you eat the F2 way.

# **F2** stand-by-soups

Select and prepare any two of the soups from the recipes on the following pages. Then try two more when stocks run low . . . and so on. Never let supplies run out. These soups can be eaten as meals, with meals or between meals. They are low enough in fat to be eaten freely. No need to count units. All are quick and easy to make. Each recipe makes sufficient for 6–8 portions so you can put some in the fridge and freeze the remainder for future use.

## Seasoning

Salt won't affect weight, but can adversely affect health, so add as little as possible. Often there's enough in the stock. Pepper? We once asked an eminent nutritionist whether he had anything against it. He answered: 'Not *yet*.' So go ahead while the going's good.

## Stock

Celeb cooks are particularly partial to Marigold Swiss Vegetable Bouillon Powder (you can get it in most supermarkets), but feel free to use any favourite vegetable stock.

## Garnishes

Chopped parsley, coriander or any other herbs will do nothing but good. Scatter them freely.

## Lemon juice

This is particularly effective in lowering the GI of a meal and a squeeze of it is good in almost any soup. Try it.

## Gadget

The world's best cooking gadget, and a blessing for soup-making, is a hand-held electric blender you can put straight into the pan to purée ingredients. It only needs rinsing under the tap. Alternatively, all these soups can be whizzed, in batches, in a blender or food processor, but this makes for more washing-up.

# Spicy Sweet Potato Soup

You can make this vegetable soup as spicy as you like by using just the curry powder, or just the ginger, or both. It is packed with bio-active veg, and even tastes delicious if you use the fast-track version below to make just about the easiest, healthy soup we know.

### MAKES 6–8 PORTIONS

- 1 large onion
- 1kg/2lb 4oz orange-fleshed sweet potatoes
- 25g/1oz fresh root ginger (optional)
- 1tbsp vegetable oil
- 1tbsp mild curry powder

- 2 litres/3½ pts of vegetable stock, hot
- Two 410g cans of cannellini beans, drained and rinsed
- 1 lemon
- salt and freshly ground black pepper
- bunch of fresh coriander (optional)

**1** Peel and roughly chop the onion and sweet potatoes. Peel the ginger (if used) and finely chop into small pieces.

**2** Heat the oil in a large saucepan, add the onion and ginger and sauté gently for 5 minutes until the onion is softened.

**3** Stir in the curry powder and cook gently for 2 minutes. Be very careful not to let the mixture burn.

**4** Add the sweet potatoes to the pan and stir to coat with the spicy onion mixture.

**5** Pour in the stock, bring to the boil, then reduce the heat, cover and cook for 20 minutes or until the sweet potatoes are tender.

**6** Blend the soup in the pan using an electric hand blender.

**7** Add the grated zest and juice from the lemon and season to taste. Stir in the cannellini beans and warm through for 5 minutes.

**8** Roughly chop the coriander, if liked, and stir into the soup.

**Fast track version** When in a hurry there's a very fast version of this soup which still tastes really good. Omit the onion, oil, ginger and coriander. Just peel the sweet potatoes, cut into small cubes and put straight into a large pan with the hot stock. Simmer for 15 minutes or until the sweet potatoes are soft. Add half the beans and the curry powder, then whizz until smooth. Add the remaining drained whole beans and cook gently for another 15 minutes. Taste for curry powder and add seasoning if needed. That's it!

# Red Lentil and Tomato Soup

Unlike some other dried pulses, lentils, which top the fibre table, do not need to be soaked before cooking. The carrots give a sweet edge to this thick, smooth soup.

## MAKES 6–8 PORTIONS

- 1 onion
- 2 medium-sized carrots
- 2 celery sticks
- 1 tbsp vegetable oil
- 200g/7oz red split lentils

- 400g can of tomatoes
- 2 litres/3½ pints of vegetable stock, hot
- 1 tbsp tomato purée
- Juice of half a lemon
- salt and freshly ground pepper

**1** Peel the onion and carrots and roughly chop them along with the celery sticks. Size isn't important as the soup is going to be puréed when the vegetables are cooked.

**2** Heat the oil in a large saucepan, add the vegetables and sauté them gently for 5 minutes until lightly coloured.

**3** Stir in the lentils, then add the tomatoes with their juice, the vegetable stock and the tomato purée. Bring to the boil, then reduce the heat, cover and simmer for 35–40 minutes until the lentils are soft.

**4** Blend the soup in the pan using an electric hand blender.

**5** Add lemon juice, salt and pepper to taste.

# Spinach Soup with Minted Peas

Healthy young leaf spinach makes a fabulous, vibrant green soup that cooks in no time at all. Adding minted peas not only boosts fibre content and gives substance to the soup but also cleverly provides a subtle mint flavour. This soup couldn't be simpler or healthier. You'll almost feel it doing you good.

## MAKES 6–8 PORTIONS

- 1 large onion
- 2 celery sticks
- 500g/1lb 2oz fresh leaf spinach, ready washed
- 1tbsp olive oil
- 1.5 litres/2¾ pints vegetable stock, hot
- 300g/11oz frozen minted peas
- juice of half a lemon
- salt and freshly ground pepper

**1** Peel the onion then roughly chop both the onion and celery.

**2** Heat the oil in a large saucepan, add the onion and celery and sauté gently for 10–15 minutes, until softened.

**3** Pour in the hot stock, bring to the boil, then add the peas and bring back to the boil again. Reduce heat and simmer gently for 2–3 minutes.

**4** Add the spinach to the pan in big handfuls, adding more as it almost immediately wilts down. Raw spinach leaves are very bulky, but quickly cook down to a small quantity, so don't be alarmed if you initially think that you are cooking far too much!

**5** As soon as all the spinach is in the pan, remove the pan from the heat – the spinach hardly needs to cook at all. Blend the soup in the pan using an electric hand blender.

**6** Stir in the lemon juice and season to taste with salt and pepper.

# Spiced Carrot and Orange Soup

Carrots, a good source of vegetable fibre, and onions, the favourite food of ultra good bifidobacteria, are the healthy basis of this delicious soup.

### MAKES 6–8 PORTIONS

- 2 large onions
- 1kg/2lb 4oz carrots
- 1 tbsp olive oil
- 1 tsp ground cumin
- 1 tsp ground coriander
- 2 litres/3½ pints vegetable stock, hot
- 2 large juicy oranges
- salt and freshly ground black pepper
- 3 tbsp chopped fresh coriander

**1** Peel and slice the onions and carrots. (Choose large carrots so there's less peeling and chopping to do.) Heat the oil in a non-stick pan and sauté the onions on a moderate heat for 5 minutes until they have softened.

**2** Stir in the spices and the carrots. Pour in the hot stock. If you like a spicy flavour you can increase the quantity of spices to 2 tsp each of cumin and coriander.

**3** Grate the zest from the oranges, taking care not to remove the white pith as this tastes bitter. Squeeze the juice from both oranges. Add the orange juice and zest to the soup. Season with pepper and salt if necessary, then bring to the boil, reduce the heat, cover and simmer for 20–25 minutes until the carrots are tender.

**4** Blend the soup in the pan using an electric hand blender.

**5** Stir in the chopped fresh coriander and taste to check seasoning. (If freezing the soup, add the fresh coriander when you come to eat the soup, for the best flavour.)

# Green Pea Soup

All the comforting thickness of a dried-pea soup with the added fresh green of frozen peas in this bio-active and filling soup.

## MAKES 6–8 PORTIONS

- 350g/12oz dried split green peas
- 1 large onion
- 1tbsp olive oil
- 2 sticks celery
- 2 carrots
- 850ml /1½ pints vegetable stock
- 400g/14oz frozen peas
- 1tbsp chopped fresh mint or 1tsp dried mint
- Salt and freshly ground pepper

**1** Put the dried split green peas in a bowl, cover with 1.15 litres/2 pints cold water and soak for 6 hours or overnight.

**2** Peel and chop the onion. Sauté in the oil in a large saucepan for 5 minutes until soft.

**3** Trim and roughly chop the celery and peel and roughly chop the carrots. Add to the pan, stir well, then add the dried split green peas and their soaking liquid and the stock.

**4** Bring to the boil. Simmer, uncovered, for an hour or until the peas are tender, skimming off the scum that rises to the surface with a large metal spoon from time to time.

**5** Add the frozen peas and mint and bring back to the boil. Simmer for about 5 minutes until the frozen peas are cooked.

**6** Blend the soup in the pan using an electric hand blender.

**7** Season to taste if necessary.

# Tex-Mex Chilli Bean Soup

A colourful soup, full of the best do-you-good veg, inspired by the flavours of chilli con carne, but without the meat.

## MAKES 6–8 PORTIONS

- 1 large onion
- 2 celery sticks
- 1 large red pepper
- 2 garlic cloves (optional)
- 1 tbsp olive oil
- 1 tsp ground cumin
- 1 tsp dried oregano
- ½ tsp chilli powder
- 1.5 litres/2¾ pints vegetable stock, hot
- 4 tbsp tomato purée
- 400g can of chopped tomatoes
- 400g can of red kidney beans
- 340g can of sweetcorn niblets

**1** Peel and finely chop the onion and celery. Cut the red pepper in half, remove the seeds and cut out the white membrane, then dice the flesh. Peel and crush the garlic, if using. (It's best not to add garlic if you plan to freeze the soup for any length of time.)

**2** Heat the olive oil in a large saucepan. Add the onion and cook gently for 5 minutes until softened. Stir in the celery, red pepper and garlic and continue to cook for a further 5 minutes.

**3** Stir in the herbs and spices, then pour in the stock and add the tomato purée and canned tomatoes with their juice. Bring to the boil, then reduce the heat, cover and simmer for 15 minutes.

**4** Drain and rinse the kidney beans and the sweetcorn, then tip them both into the pan. Simmer for 5–10 minutes (they don't need cooking, just heating through).

**5** No need to blend the soup, but if you choose to do so blend for just a few seconds in the pan using an electric hand blender, so that it is lightly thickened but most of the beans and vegetables are still in chunks. Season to taste if you like, but you will probably find this unnecessary.

# **F2** stand-by salads

Select and prepare any two of the following. All these salads keep well in covered containers in the fridge for several days. They give a major boost to fibre and resistant starch intake, stimulating healthy bio-action, helping to speed weight loss and keep blood sugar levels on an even keel.

Aim to keep two salads on stand-by in the fridge. They can be used as side salads with meals or as a meal in themselves, perhaps with 'a little something' from our Easy Meal suggestions.

## Dressings

Most of these recipes include fat-free or low-fat dressings for which fat units are included in the total. Where a vinaigrette (French) dressing is indicated, either choose a 'low-fat' or 'fat-free' shop-bought product, make your own 'two-to-one' (two tablespoons of oil to one of vinegar) version or try **Very Vinaigeryette** on page 120. Fat units for all these alternatives are given on page 155.

The oils used in salad dressings are the beneficial kind. But curtail the quantity and steer clear of very oily dressings because of their high calorie content. With some salads you might find that a splash of balsamic vinegar, less sharp than other vinegars, is acceptable on its own as a fat-free dressing.

# Carrot, Almond and Raisin Salad

**FAT UNITS**

**0**

Make this salad your first choice. It has the advantages of being remarkably easy to make, lasting well in the fridge and perfectly partnering any of the other essential salads. Big bonus: it needs no dressing other than GI-lowering lemon juice and offers a remarkable range of health benefits. Almonds have been named by scientists as among those foods 'most likely to prolong life'. No need to count the fat units for the small quantity in this otherwise fat-free dish. Carrots and lemon juice contain some of the most powerful cancer-preventing nutrients.

### MAKES 4–6 PORTIONS

- 5 medium-sized carrots
- 25g/1oz toasted flaked almonds
- 25g/1oz currants or raisins
- juice of 1 small lemon

**1** Peel and coarsely grate the carrots. Tip into a bowl or lidded plastic container.

**2** Flaked almonds can be bought ready-toasted, but if you need to toast your own scatter them on the base of a grill pan or baking sheet and toast under a hot grill until golden. This only takes about 30 seconds so keep an eye on them or they will burn. It saves time to toast a whole packet in one go and store the surplus in an airtight jar.

**3** Add the toasted almonds and raisins/currants to the carrots, sprinkle over the lemon juice and toss well. Cover and keep in the fridge.

**Variation** If you have time to peel and pith an orange and chop the segments into chunky pieces (after removing any tough membranes) it makes a lovely fruity addition to this salad.

# Butter Bean Salad with Spring Onions and Maple Mustard Dressing

This delicious and very easy salad is adapted from one of our favourite cookery books, *Vegetarian Express* (Cassell). We've included it by kind permission of queen of the veggie cooks, Rose Elliot. Rose serves it warm on a heap of green salad leaves. That way it makes a wonderful and 'very **F2**' light lunch, maybe after a bowl of **F2** soup.

You can also enjoy it cold as a stand-by salad. The dressing is relatively low in fat compared to most. If this becomes one of your regular favourites, we suggest you make sufficient dressing for four servings and store in a jar in the fridge. The salad is put together so quickly that it's hardly worth pre-preparing.

### MAKES 2 GENEROUS PORTIONS

- 425g can butter beans
- 2 tbsp maple syrup
- 1 tbsp Dijon mustard
- 1 tbsp balsamic vinegar
- 1 tbsp olive oil
- 6 spring onions, chopped
- 2–3 tbsp chopped fresh coriander (optional)
- Salad leaves

**1** Place the butter beans and their liquid in a saucepan and warm over a moderate heat for about 5 minutes until heated through.

**2** Meanwhile mix together the maple syrup, mustard, balsamic vinegar and olive oil.

**3** Drain the beans and mix gently with the maple-syrup dressing, the spring onions and the chopped coriander. Spoon half the quantity on to a base of salad leaves and serve.

**4** Store the remaining half in a covered container in the fridge to be eaten cold, heaped on to crisp green salad leaves, as a stand-by salad.

# Bean, Sweetcorn and Red Pepper Salad

This excellent and 'moreish' salad is packed with veg of outstanding value for positive health. It calls out for vinaigrette (French) dressing, so choose one of the options. The fat units in a serving will depend on your choice – the veg are virtually fat-free.

## MAKES 4–6 PORTIONS

- 300g can cannellini or red kidney beans
- 340g can sweetcorn
- Half a medium-sized onion
- 1 large red pepper
- 3–4 tbsp fresh coriander, chopped

**1** Drain the beans and sweetcorn. Tip into a large bowl or lidded plastic container.

**2** Peel and finely chop the onion. Halve the pepper, remove seeds and membranes, then dice. Mix all ingredients.

**3** Drizzle over the dressing and toss well, then add the coriander and toss again.

**Variation** For a spicy note you can add a fresh red chilli to this salad. Cut it in half and remove the seeds, taking care not to touch your face. Finely chop the chilli and add to the salad with the pepper. Wash your hands thoroughly afterwards.

# Spicy Chickpeas with Rich Tomato Dressing

FAT UNITS
1½

Like the Butter Bean Salad, this dish can start as a hot meal – we've included it among the baked potato Easy Meal suggestions. The remainder, with crunchy celery and sweetcorn added, can be stored in the fridge as a stand-by salad. Chickpeas are a great source of fibre, and this salad, in its own spicy low-fat tomato sauce, needs no added dressing.

## MAKES 4 PORTIONS

- 1 medium onion
- 1 tbsp vegetable oil
- 1 tbsp mild or medium curry powder
- 700g jar passata
- 1 tbsp mango chutney
- 1 tbsp lemon juice
- 400g can chickpeas, drained
- 2–3 celery sticks
- 200g can sweetcorn, drained

**1** Chop the onion into quite small dice. Heat the oil in a non-stick pan then sauté the onion on a gentle heat for 5 minutes, until softened. Stir in the curry powder and cook gently for 5 minutes more, taking care not to allow the powder to burn.

**2** Add the passata to the pan with the chutney and lemon juice. Bring to the boil, then reduce the heat, add the chickpeas and cook gently for 10 minutes. One portion could be served hot with a baked potato and green veg as a main meal.

**3** To make a stand-by salad simply allow the remainder to cool, then mix in the sliced celery and sweetcorn. Cover and keep chilled.

# Quick Pasta Salad with Salsa Dressing

Cold pasta is one of the very best sources of 'retrograded starch'. This is even more effective than other fibre components in stimulating good bacteria to produce health-protective substances. Wholewheat pasta is a superfood for all aspects of health and weight control – but cold wholewheat pasta is best of all. This shortcut recipe makes pasta salad very easy to make, while avoiding the large quantity of oily dressing in shop-bought versions.

## MAKES 4–6 PORTIONS

- 200g/7oz wholewheat pasta shells or shapes

- 375g jar of salsa dip (mild or hot) or two 170g cartons of chilled salsa dip
- 200g can sweetcorn, drained
- ¼ cucumber, diced

**1** Cook the pasta until al dente (just tender) according to packet instructions. Drain, rinse and drain thoroughly again. Tip into a large bowl or lidded plastic container.

**2** Add the salsa dip to the pasta and stir well to coat all the shells.

**3** Mix in the sweetcorn and cucumber. Cover and chill. Eat within 3 days.

**Variations** Diced green, red or yellow pepper could be used in place of the cucumber. You could also stir in some halved cherry tomatoes or a few stoned olives. Chopped fresh herbs, such as basil or chives, would be delicious added just before serving.

# Puy Lentil and Cranberry Salad

**FAT**
UNITS
**2**

This salad takes just a little longer to make but is worth the effort. Lentils are particularly high in fibre and don't cause flatulence, as other legumes can tend to do until you get used to them. We've adapted this recipe from an idea in Leon Lewis's *More Vegetarian Dinner Parties* (Free Range Publishing). It was gobbled up to the last lentil at a recent party of our own. The dried cranberries, which can be bought in packets in most supermarkets, add a delicious and unusual note as well as valuable nutrients. This recipe makes a generous quantity, but it is certainly good enough to share.

## MAKES 6–8 PORTIONS

- 250g/9oz puy lentils
- 750ml vegetable stock (Marigold Swiss Vegetable Bouillon is good)
- 1 carrot, finely chopped
- 1 onion, finely chopped
- 2 celery sticks, finely chopped
- 1 large courgette, finely chopped
- 75g packet of dried cranberries
- 1tbsp sunflower oil

### FOR THE DRESSING:
- 2 tbsp extra virgin olive oil
- 1tbsp balsamic vinegar
- 2–3 garlic cloves
- salt and freshly ground black pepper
- 3 tbsp chopped fresh parsley

**1** Rinse the lentils in a sieve, then put them in a saucepan and pour on the hot stock. Bring to the boil, then reduce the heat and cook gently for 15–20 minutes until the lentils are just tender.

**2** Meanwhile heat the sunflower oil in a frying pan, add the chopped vegetables and sauté gently for 10 minutes until softened.

**3** Put the olive oil and vinegar in a screw-top jar, crush in the garlic, season and shake well to make the dressing.

**4** Combine the drained lentils, vegetables, cranberries and chopped parsley in a large bowl. Stir in the dressing. Cool, cover and keep in the fridge.

**Variation** A red pepper, roasted until soft, peeled, de-seeded and cut into thin slices (another inspiration from Leon) is a delicious garnish for this salad.

# Bulgar Wheat, Apricot and Chickpea Salad

**FAT**
UNITS
**0**

Again a vinaigrette dressing would be best. Choose from the options given on pages 120–1, adding the appropriate number of fat units. All other ingredients are virtually fat-free.

### MAKES 4–6 PORTIONS

- 200g/7oz bulgar wheat
- 400g can chickpeas
- 100g/3½ oz dried ready-to-eat apricots
- 2 celery sticks
- 4 spring onions
- 2 pieces Chinese stem ginger, drained of syrup
- 2 tbsp chopped fresh parsley or mint (optional)
- salt and freshly ground black pepper

**1** Tip the bulgar wheat into a large bowl and pour over 500ml/ 18fl oz boiling water, to cover. Stir then leave to soak for about 20 minutes until the water is absorbed. The absorbency can vary – if there's water left in the bowl drain the bulgar in a sieve.

**2** Drain the chickpeas and add to the bulgar. Chop the apricots, thinly slice the celery and spring onions, then toss them all into the salad.

**3** Finely chop the ginger, add it to the dressing in a screw-top jar and shake well. Drizzle over the salad and toss through. Add seasoning, parsley or mint to taste and toss again, then cover and keep in the fridge.

# VERY VINAIGERYETTE

This is my own low-fat version of vinaigrette – and rates as something of a culinary crime, I suspect. Search as you will in any cookery book (I have), you won't find it. Yet, being very conscious of the staggering calorie content of oil, this is the 'vinaigrette' I've been making for years, even serving to guests. And, much to my surprise, I've had almost as many compliments about it – even, would you believe it, recipe requests – as I've had cold suppers.

Proper cooks, of course, wouldn't dream of using less than treble the quantity of oil to that of vinegar. Me? More or less half and half. I use a mix of sunflower and olive oil and wine vinegar. Into this goes just a little salt, black pepper, a generous dollop of Dijon mustard and lots of crushed garlic.

While in confessional mode, I might as well admit that I have been known to use that ready-crushed garlic from a bottle, and – oh, what the hell! – I shake it all up in a jar ages before a meal rather than (sorry, Delia!) freshly crushing, mixing and blending at the last minute with pestle and mortar while the dog is barking at the throats of anxiously arriving guests. But brace yourself, we are yet to come to the *real* culinary crime. Gordon Ramsay would no doubt rate it a knifing offence. My final ingredient is a good teaspoon of sugar. OK, if it's a biggish jar, even two good teaspoons of sugar.

Apart from the relief of getting that off my chest, I have good reason for confiding. Sugar has only half the calories of oil. Added (as it never is by stylish cooks) to vinaigrette it takes the sharpness off this mix, which contains a high content of GI-lowering vinegar and a relatively low content of high-calorie oil.

Why not try it? You might hate it. But if not you will have a lower-calorie homemade vinaigrette that you can use more freely than most and might even enjoy as much as I do. Count 2½ fat units per tablespoon.

## Alternative version

My weight-conscious home-economist friend Glynis McGuinness makes her own 'very vinaigeryette' with equal amounts of balsamic vinegar (less sharp than wine vinegar) and oil, a small amount of clear honey and a tiny amount of Dijon mustard. Like me, she has come to find classic vinaigrette 'too oily for my taste'.

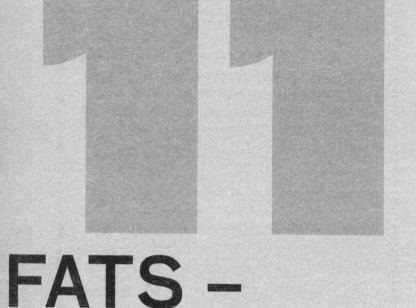

# FATS –
# THE FACTS

# CRUCIAL INFO FOR WEIGHT AND HEALTH!

## All oils and fats are fattening, very fattening

All supply more than 200 calories an ounce – twice as many as sugar, for instance, or any other fat-free food. There are a whopping 130 calories in just one tablespoon of oil.

Don't make the common mistake of thinking that healthier fats, such as olive oil, are any less fattening than other fats.

## All fatty foods are fattening too

Fats lurk, often unsuspected, in all those battered and breadcrumbed foods, many ready-meals and fast-food restaurant meals, cheesy dishes, crisps, dips, pastry products, biscuits, cakes, chips, chocs, creamy soups, oily sauces, mayonnaise-rich sandwiches . . . the list is endless. We're under fat attack from every direction.

Hidden fats can even come in healthy, natural foods. Nuts and seeds, for instance, though packed with healthy nutrients, are rich in oil. You can't afford to eat too many if you want to lose weight.

## Fats and health

There are three types of fat: saturated, polyunsaturated and monounsaturated. All fats are a mixture of these, but health dangers or benefits are determined by which type predominates, and in some cases by food-manufacturing processes.

Health authorities recommend that we eat less fat overall and focus on the healthier kind.

# The bad fats

The less we eat of these the better!

## Saturated fats

● Dairy and meat products are the major source of saturated fat in the Western diet. Products made from whole milk or cream, such as butter, dairy ice-creams and most cheeses, are particularly rich sources.

● Coconut and palm oils (often called tropical oils), used in some canned and processed foods, are also mainly saturated. Avoid these and 'blended vegetable oils', which often contain them.

For years health experts have rated saturated fat, which raises cholesterol in the blood, the single greatest danger in the Western diet. A truly vast quantity of evidence links it with clogging the arteries with plaque, which impedes blood flow to the heart and brain, leading to heart disease and strokes.

Growing evidence also links saturated fat with breast and prostate cancer. Initial findings from the most definitive diet-and-cancer study ever conducted, the European Prospective Investigation into Cancer and Nutrition, indicate that women who eat too much dairy fat and meat double their breast-cancer risk. This current study of half a million people in ten European countries has real import, unlike so many of the small or badly designed studies publicized these days. Other recent studies reveal that breast cancer has doubled in Japan since the younger generation adopted a Western diet.

## Trans fats

● These lurk in some margarines and fat spreads, in many readymade goods such as biscuits, cakes and crisps, and in most deep-fried fast foods.

Trans fats are made when manufacturers solidify vegetable oils to make margarine by using hydrogen. They are as dangerously artery-clogging as saturated fats, possibly even more so.

If the ingredients list on a food label contains the word 'hydrogenated', the product is likely to contain trans fats. Avoid margarine-type spreads which state 'hydrogenated' or 'partially hydrogenated'. Choose those like Flora on which the labels state 'no trans fats' or 'non hydrogenated'.

Hydrogenated oils are used in so many manufactured foods that they are very hard to avoid completely. But **F2**'s Fat and Calorie Controller will prove a boon in showing you how to ration or screen out those with a high content.

# The good fats

Focus on these fats – particularly when you are rationing fats to weight-loss level.

# Polyunsaturated fats supplying essential Omega 3 fatty acids

● Richest sources are oily fish – mackerel, herring, sardines, anchovies, tuna, trout and salmon. Wild fish tends to be a better source than farmed fish.

● Richest plant sources are flaxseeds, walnuts and their oils.

● Omega 3 free-range eggs are now sold in major stores and one egg can provide a half to two-thirds of the recommended daily amount of Omega 3.

The polyunsaturated fats are not cholesterol-raising or artery-clogging and we need a small quantity of them to supply essential fatty acids. There are two types of these, Omega 3 and Omega 6. We're unlikely to go short of Omega 6, but nowadays we tend not to eat enough Omega 3. This is suspected of being a causal factor in heart and other major health problems.

As a result of raised awareness, Omega 3 eggs – probably the easiest way to ensure you get enough of this nutrient – have become widely available in the supermarkets, and you can choose from a whole range of flaxseed oils, or, better still, flaxseeds themselves, in health-food shops. But remember that even oil rich in Omega 3 is high in calories. Choose fish in preference to meat, but go easy on oily fish, both on account of the calorie score and concerns about its content of potentially harmful substances called dioxins.

# Monounsaturated fats

● Richest sources are olive oil, rapeseed oil (canola), peanut oil and the oil in avocados.

Monounsaturated fats are even more healthy than poly-unsaturated fats. They lower cholesterol to the same extent but also distribute it in the blood in a healthier way.

Olive oil has a particularly high content of monounsat-urates. Rapeseed oil is almost as good. The widespread use of olive oil, along with low meat and dairy intake and the consumption of large quantities of fruit, veg, grains and fish, lies behind the famed health benefits of Mediterranean diets.

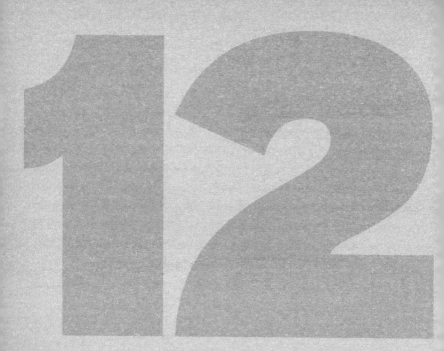

# 12
# THE FAT AND CALORIE CONTROLLER

THIS CHART IS about to become your figure's best friend. It will tell you which foods were making you overweight (stand by for shocks), which to choose to get slim, and which to go easy on in the future.

All highly fattening foods are fatty foods. It's that fat – more than twice as high in calories as anything else – that zooms up calorie intake to weight-gain levels. And there's so much of it, most of it invisible and unsuspected, in so many of today's ready-mades. That's why, as well as guiding you to the right foods for healthy weight loss, the **F2** chart includes some what-not-to-eat warning items.

● Eat freely from the virtually fat-free vegetables, fruit and grain-based foods recommended in the **F2** rules.

● Allow yourself up to 10 units a day from the fat-containing foods in this chart and watch your own surplus fat simply melt away.

# ● AVOCADO PEARS

Avocado oil is healthy oil but, when dieting to shed weight, sometimes you can have too much of a good thing. This is the only fruit you'll need to limit on **F2**. Other fruit and veg are virtually fat-free.

**HALF SMALL AVOCADO**
(150g/5oz weighed whole with skin and stone) ...................**3½**

**HALF MEDIUM AVOCADO**
(200g/7oz weighed whole as above)........................................**4**

**HALF LARGE AVOCADO**
(275g/10oz weighed whole as above) .....................................**6**

**GUACAMOLE,** per 25g/1oz ....**2**

**GUACAMOLE,** per rounded
teaspoon ......................................**1**

**GUACAMOLE,** per 170g pot .**11**

**REDUCED-FAT GUACAMOLE,**
per 25g/1oz..............................**1**

**REDUCED-FAT GUACAMOLE,**
per rounded teaspoon ...........**½**

**REDUCED-FAT GUACAMOLE,**
per 170g pot ........................**6½**

# ● BISCUITS

Buy yourself a packet of favourite biscuits, keep them in the kitchen, try not to eat them. Now just how smart is that? Yet rather than side-stepping temptation, dieters often feel a kamikaze urge to fling themselves in its path. **F2** will change your eating preferences, but it doesn't happen overnight. Meanwhile, if biscuits are what rocks your boat, deploy those few minutes it takes to resist buying them in the shop rather than whole days trying to resist eating them once they're in the house. Here are the fat units to count if you accept a biscuit or two in a safer public situation. Most contain unhealthy trans or saturated fats, so limit them to two a day, max.

**Fat units are given per biscuit unless otherwise stated.**

## SWEET BISCUITS

BISCOTTI ...................................**2**

BOURBON CREAM................**1**

SMALL CHOCOLATE CHIP
AND NUT COOKIE ..............**1**

CHOCOLATE FINGER ..........**½**

COCONUT RING ....................**1**

CUSTARD CREAM..................**1**

DIGESTIVE, CHOCOLATE,
large .....................................**1½**

DIGESTIVE, PLAIN, large ......**1**

SMALL FRUIT

  SHORTCAKE .........................**1**

GINGER NUT ...........................½

ICED SHORTIE ......................½

JAFFA CAKE ...........................½

JAM SANDWICH CREAM......**1**

LINCOLN, 2 biscuits................½

MORNING COFFEE,

  2 biscuits...............................½

NICE ...........................................½

PETIT BEURRE .....................½

RICH TEA...............................½

## SAVOURY BISCUITS

BREAD STICKS, 3 sticks ......½

BUTTER PUFF .......................**1**

CREAM CRACKER ...............½

OATCAKE ...............................**1**

WATER BISCUIT, 2 biscuits ..½

## ● BUTTER AND MARGARINE-TYPE SPREADS

Do you own a 5ml measuring teaspoon? No? Then on your bike. Buy one before you even begin **F2**, for reasons obvious from the figures below. When it comes to undiluted fat, even a scraping counts in calories. Precision is vital. We've given fat units per 25g/1oz and per level – note that 'level' – teaspoon. All brands of products, including the supermarkets' own brands, supply the same number of fat units as those below. Turn to page 147 for equally nasty figures for oils.

BUTTER (including types
labelled 'spreadable')
per 25g/1oz ............................**8**
per level teaspoon .............**1½**

GHEE per 25g/1oz ................**10**
per level teaspoon .............**1½**

LOW-FAT SPREADS (e.g. Flora
Light, Gold, Benecol Light) per
25g/1oz................................**3½**
per level teaspoon.................½

MARGARINE, block or soft per
25g/1oz ...................................**8**
per level teaspoon ..............**1½**

OLIVE-OIL-BASED SPREADS
(e.g. Olivio) per 25g/1oz..........**6**
per level teaspoon ..................**1**

SUNFLOWER SPREAD per
25g/1oz ...................................**6**
per level teaspoon ..................**1**

# ● CAKES

The same warnings apply as for biscuits. Buy a whole big cake or a packet of favourite individual cakes and sooner or later you'll be sneaking downstairs again (*don't think we weren't watching!*) in those wee small hours of the night. If cakes are on your hard-to-resist list buy only a single individual cake to cope with what, for many women, might be a strong 'time of the month' craving. The quantity you buy is the quantity you'll eat (*Oh yes you will!*). And avert your eyes from those deceptively healthy-looking oaty flapjacks on sale in shops, cafés, trains, trolleys, kiosks, petrol stations . . . just about everywhere, these days, bar public loos.

**Fat units given per average-sized cake.**

| | |
|---|---|
| ALMOND SLICE OR | FLAKE CAKE ...........................2 |
| BAKEWELL SLICE..................2 | FLAPJACK (115g/4oz) ............9 |
| APPLE PIE ..............................3 | FRENCH FANCY .....................1 |
| CHOCOLATE-COATED MINI | JAM DOUGHNUT ..................4 |
| ROLL ......................................2 | JAM TART ............................1½ |
| SMALL CHOCOLATE OR | MINCE PIE............................3½ |
| LEMON CUP CAKE ............½ | VIENNESE WHIRL .................3 |

# ● CHEESE

Most cheese is exceedingly high in fat. Worse – it is one of the main sources of health-threatening saturated fat which raises bad cholesterol. Few fully realize just how major a role it can play in weight and heart problems. Choose only the low-fat cheeses. Eat other cheeses only in small quantities, or as an occasional treat. If they are on your hard-to-resist list buy them only in those tiny 1oz packs now conveniently on sale. Go for the stronger flavours to get more eating satisfaction from less.

**Fat units are given per 25g/1oz unless otherwise stated.**

| | |
|---|---|
| BAVARIAN SMOKED | 2½ |
| BRIE | 3 |
| BOURSIN | 4 |
| CAERPHILLY | 3 |
| CAMEMBERT | 2½ |
| CHEDDAR | 3½ |
| CHEESE SPREAD | 2½ |
| CHEESE SPREAD per triangle | ½ |
| CHESHIRE | 3 |
| COTTAGE CHEESE | ½ |
| COTTAGE CHEESE, per 225g carton | 3½ |
| COTTAGE CHEESE, reduced fat, per 75g/3oz | ½ |
| COTTAGE CHEESE, reduced fat, per 225g carton | 1 |
| DANISH BLUE | 3 |
| DOLCELATTE | 3½ |
| EDAM | 2½ |
| FETA | 2 |
| GOAT'S CHEESE, soft with white rind | 2½ |
| GORGONZOLA | 3 |
| GOUDA | 3 |
| GRUYERE | 3 |
| HALOUMI | 2½ |
| LANCASHIRE | 3 |
| MASCARPONE | 3½ |
| MOZZARELLA | 2 |
| MOZZARELLA, reduced fat or 'light' | 1 |
| MOZZARELLA, per 125g/4½oz ball | 9 |
| PARMESAN | 3½ |
| RED LEICESTER | 3½ |
| RICOTTA | 1 |
| SOFT CHEESE, full fat | 3 |
| SOFT CHEESE, half fat | 1½ |
| SOFT CHEESE, less than 10 per cent fat | ½ |
| STILTON, blue | 3½ |
| WENSLEYDALE | 3 |

## ● CHOCOLATE

Chocolate cravings can be highly powerful. No normal chocolate-loving woman can trust herself with favourite chocolates in the house. Don't even try. Avoid boxes and multi-packs. If given a box of chocs (as you almost certainly will be as you are seen to lose weight – people are funny like that!), pass it on *instantly* to someone thin. Or to someone you don't like.

The bars we've listed below can be bought individually and eaten to satisfy a craving without turning it into a binge. Counted as part of your 10 daily units they won't even damage your diet. But eat them as infrequently as possible. Chocolate has an addictive quality and the more often you eat it the more

often you want it. Regard these as emergency buys.
**Fat units are given per bar or bag.**

## CADBURY'S

| | |
|---|---|
| BUBBLY BAR | **3½** |
| BUTTONS, small bag | **3½** |
| CHOCOLATE CREAM BAR | **2½** |
| CREME EGG | **2½** |
| CRUNCHIE | **2½** |
| DIPPED FLAKE | **5** |
| FLAKE | **3½** |
| ORANGE CREAM | **2½** |
| PEPPERMINT CREAM | **2½** |
| SNOWFLAKE | **4** |
| TURKISH DELIGHT | **1½** |
| WAFER BAR | **4½** |

## MARS

| | |
|---|---|
| MILKY WAY | **1½** |
| GALAXY RIPPLE | **3½** |
| MALTESERS, 37g pack | **3** |

## NESTLÉ

| | |
|---|---|
| AERO, chunky bar | **4** |
| KIT KAT, 2 finger | **2** |
| KIT KAT, Orange Editions | **3½** |

## ● CREAM

Think of cream, as nutritionists do, as 'the fat of the milk' and one of our main sources of health-threatening saturated fat. Not enough to put you off? Then maybe the following figures, each for the modest quantity that can be contained in a 15ml level tablespoon, will help.

| | |
|---|---|
| CLOTTED CREAM | **3½** |
| CREME FRAICHE | **2** |
| CREME FRAICHE, reduced fat | **1** |
| DOUBLE CREAM | **3** |
| SINGLE CREAM | **1** |
| SOURED CREAM | **1** |
| WHIPPING CREAM | **2** |

## ● DELI AND DIPS

There are some handy dieting items on the deli counter. Some dangerous ones, too. Bad bacteria love to shop there for deli meats – just the ammunition they need to overwhelm your good bacteria. Quorn slices (page 157) are an alternative – not bad if you lash on the pickle. Many a meat pie or deli meat item is

eaten largely in response to an urge for Branston or the like, and
McDonald's would close (I think I could just about live with that!)
if all their relishes and sauces were banned.

CHINESE VEGETABLE
SPRING ROLLS, Per roll,
average, 25g/1oz .....................**1**
Per roll, large, 40g/1½oz ....**1½**

## OLIVES
WHOLE OLIVES, per 25g/1oz
(approx 6 olives).........................**1**
OLIVE TAPENADE, per
25g/1oz ...................................**1**
OLIVE TAPENADE, per level
tablespoon .............................**½**

## SALSA
SALSA (tomato or red pepper)
per 200g pot ...........................**1**

## SCOTCH EGGS
SCOTCH EGG, 115g/4oz ....**7½**

PICNIC EGG OR SNACK
EGG, 40g/1½oz ..................**3½**
MINI EGGS, 20g/¾oz ..........**1½**
MINI EGG BITES, 15g/½oz ....**1**

## STUFFED VINE LEAVES
Well drained of oil, each
(approx 50g/2oz) ...................**1**

## SUN DRIED TOMATOES
Per tomato, well drained........**½**

## SUNBLUSH TOMATOES
Well drained and wiped of oil,
per 25g/1oz..............................**½**
TARAMASALATA Per 25g/
1oz ........................................**4½**
Per 170g pot ........................**28**

## ● EGGS
MEDIUM-SIZED EGGS,
each .........................................**2**

LARGE EGGS, each ............**2½**

## ● EGG NOODLES
READY-TO-STIR-FRY
NOODLES, per 25g/1oz ......**½**

DRY EGG NOODLES, per
25g/1oz ..................................**1**

# ● FISH

White fish, very low in fatty calories, can make the ideal dieting meal. Unless, of course, the chip shop fries it in batter – a full daily ration of 10 fat units in that little lot! Oily fish is a rich source of the healthy Omega 3 fatty acids you need – but also of the calories you don't. Keep portions small while slimming.

Choose your fish with discretion with this guide and add units for any fat or oil used in cooking:

## WHITE FISH
**Fat units are given for a whole fresh or frozen raw fillet weighing an average 175g/6oz.**

COD OR HADDOCK, fresh or smoked, per portion ................½

MONKFISH, per portion ........½

HALIBUT OR SEA BASS, per portion ..........................1½

PLAICE, DOVER SOLE OR LEMON SOLE, per portion......1

## OILY FISH

These fish are very much higher in fatty calories so units are given per 25g/1oz of fresh or frozen fillet unless otherwise stated, *not* for a whole portion as for the white fish above. Include some in your diet for beneficial fats, but keep portions small. When possible, choose wild or organic fish.

HERRING, weighed raw (with bones) ...................................1½

HERRING, cured ....................½

KIPPER FILLET ......................2

MACKEREL, weighed raw (whole fish) ..........................1½

MACKEREL, smoked fillet ......3

SALMON STEAK, weighed raw ...........................................1

SALMON, honey roast flakes ..1

SALMON, smoked .................½

SALMON, gravalax with dill sauce, per 75g/3oz portion ......3

SARDINES, fresh whole weighed raw ..........................½

TROUT FILLET, fresh or smoked ..................................½

TROUT, per whole 225g/ 8oz fish....................................3

TUNA STEAK, weighed raw ..½

## CANNED FISH

Always drain off any oil, using kitchen tissue to absorb as much as possible. Fat units are given for the whole contents of a can, drained of fat where applicable, unless otherwise stated.

Nasty shocks department: note how mackerel, already pretty high in fatty calories in itself, gets alarmingly high when canned in rich sauces.

ANCHOVIES, per two fillets....½

CRAB, white meat only, canned
in brine, 200g ........................½

DRESSED CRAB, 43g ............**1**

MACKEREL FILLETS in brine,
125g ........................................**5**
in curry sauce,125g ............**7½**
in hot chilli dressing,125g ....**12**
in mustard sauce,125g........**7½**
in rich, spicy tomato sauce,
125g ........................................**6**

PRESSED COD ROE, 200g....**3**

SALMON, PINK, 105g ............**2**

SALMON, RED, 105g ..........**2½**

SARDINES CANNED IN OIL,
per sardine ..............................**2**

SARDINES CANNED IN
BRINE, per sardine ................**1**

SARDINES CANNED IN
TOMATO SAUCE, per
sardine ..................................**1½**

SARDINES, BONELESS IN
OIL, 95g ..............................**3½**

SILD IN OIL, 110g ................**5**

SILD IN TOMATO SAUCE,
110g ........................................**5**

SKIPPERS IN TOMATO
SAUCE, 106g ........................**5**

SOFT HERRING ROE, 125g..½

TUNA CANNED IN OIL, 100g..**2**

TUNA IN BRINE, 200g ..........½

TUNA, LIGHT SLICES
CANNED IN OIL, 120g ......**1½**

## GOLDEN COATED FISH

These days a great deal of fish is sold ready-coated in fat-containing breadcrumbs or batter. Count the following units if, occasionally (no crime if only 'from time to time') you choose this more calorie-costly way of eating fish. No extra fat need be used in cooking these products.

COD, FRIED IN BATTER, from
fish and chip shop, medium
portion ..................................**10**

COD OR HADDOCK STEAK
IN BATTER, frozen, 100g/
3½oz ........................................**5**

COD OR HADDOCK STEAK
  IN BREADCRUMBS, frozen,
  100g/3½oz .........................**3½**

COD OR HADDOCK FILLET
  IN BREADCRUMBS, 115g/
  4oz ......................................**3½**

COD OR HADDOCK FISH
  CAKE, each ........................**1½**

COD OR HADDOCK FILLET
  FISH FINGER, each .............**1**

LEMON SOLE GOUJONS, per
  115g/4oz ...............................**5**

PLAICE FILLET IN BREAD-
  CRUMBS, 115g/4oz ..............**6**

## POPULAR FROZEN FISH STEAKS IN SAUCE
**Fat units are given per pouch for these convenience meals.**

COD IN BUTTER SAUCE,
  150g .....................................**1½**

COD IN PARSLEY SAUCE,
  150g.......................................**2**

HADDOCK IN LEEK AND
  CHEESE SAUCE, 175g ....**2½**

SALMON FILLET IN DILL
  SAUCE, 175g .......................**3**

See page 156 for shellfish and seafood.

## ● HOLLANDAISE SAUCE
Very buttery and now temptingly available ready-made. Hold the Eggs Benedict for a special treat when you are slim enough to celebrate.
Per level tablespoon .............**3½**

## ● HOUMOUS
While a little houmous can be a very good thing, a lot, as with many good things, is not. Houmous is made from fibre-rich chick peas, healthy garlic and sesame seeds, but also a large quantity of oil. Don't let that put you off. Just think in terms of teaspoons rather than tablespoons of houmous. And always choose the brands labelled low-fat or less fat. Used in small quantities, houmous can be a helpful and versatile part of your

diet, and the oils it contains are of the beneficial kind – not saturated. Spread it sparingly on your wholemeal toast, for instance, or instead of butter-type spreads in a sandwich. Added flavours such as roasted red pepper will make no significant difference to the fat units below.

**ORDINARY FULL-FAT HOUMOUS:**

per 25g/1oz ...........................**3**

per rounded teaspoon ............**1**

**REDUCED-FAT HOUMOUS**

per 25g/1oz ........................**1½**

per rounded teaspoon ..........**½**

## ● ICE-CREAM

Ice-creams can figure among both the lowest-calorie and highest-calorie desserts, depending on their dairy cream content. This puts luxury brands out of court for dieting. Sorry about that. But some of the lower-calorie versions taste fine with raspberries, strawberries and blueberries, the healthiest way to eat them. So does a really good dairy-free 'ice cream' called Swedish Glace which you will find in 50p-shaped containers in Holland & Barrett and some supermarkets.

But you know yourself, and if a large tub of ice-cream presents an irresistible temptation, if you kid yourself that an enormous scoop is average, that 'just a lick' doesn't count, and suffer eating-amnesia about just how many licks you've had, better buy only individual-sized ices.

Best buys for low content of fatty calories include ice-cream and water-ice combinations such as Solero, Strawberry Fruit Double, Starburst and the supermarkets' own brands of basic choc ices, which are smaller and lower cal than luxury brands. There are also two low-fat ranges, Weight Watchers and The Skinny Cow.

Water ices, which are fat-free, can be enjoyed in moderation on F2. Let's say no more than one a day.

## BASIC SUPERMARKET MULTI-PORTION TUBS
**Per 75g/3oz portion – 2 good scoops**
VANILLA ICE CREAM ............**2**
CORNISH ICE CREAM ..........**3**

## SWEDISH GLACE MULTI-PORTION TUBS
VANILLA OR CHOCOLATE,
  per 750ml tub .......................**14**
  per 75g/3oz portion (2 good
  scoops)...............................**2½**

## BASIC SUPERMARKET OWN-BRAND CHOC ICES
**Per choc ice**
DARK OR LIGHT CHOC
  ICE .....................................**3½**

## CADBURY'S
**Per individual piece**
CRUNCHIE .........................**4½**
DAIRY MILK .......................**3½**
FLAKE 99.............................**4½**
FLAKE 99 WITH
  STRAWBERRY......................**4**
FRUIT AND NUT ...................**3**
MINT CHIPS .......................**4½**
MINT CONE ...........................**3**
TURKISH BAR .......................**6**

## DEL MONTE
**Per individual piece**
STRAWBERRY FRUIT
  DOUBLE................................**½**

## GREEN & BLACK
**Per 100ml tub**
CHOCOLATE.......................**3½**
CHOCOLATE AND
  ORANGE ...........................**3½**
DARK TOFFEE.......................**3**
VANILLA..............................**3½**

## HILL STATION
**Per 100ml tub**
BANANA MUSCOVADO......**3½**
MANGO AND LIME ...............**4**
VANILLA..............................**4½**

## MARS
**Per individual piece**
GALAXY VANILLA
  HEAVEN..............................**4½**
MARS..................................**3½**
STARBURST ...........................**1**

## THE SKINNY COW
**Per individual piece**
CHOCOLATE FUDGE STICK**½**
COOKIES 'N' CREAM
  STICK...................................**½**
MINT CHOC STICK...............**½**

RASPBERRY AND VANILLA
   CONE ....................................**1**
VERY BERRY STICK..............½

## WALL'S
**Per individual piece**
CORNETTO CLASSICO......**4½**
MAGNUM CLASSIC............**5½**
MAGNUM LIGHT ................**3½**
SOLERO EXOTIC....................**1**

VANILLA TUB, 105ml ..........**1½**

## WEIGHT WATCHERS
**Per individual piece**
CHOCOLATE ORANGE
   SUNDAE ................................**1**
DOUBLE CHOCOLATE
   BROWNIE..............................**1**
STRAWBERRY AND VANILLA
   SUNDAE ................................**1**

## ● INDIAN ITEMS

Regard Indian meals as 'add-ons' rather than 'take-aways'
where your figure is concerned. Same applies to deli items such
as onion bhajis. There's a great deal of hidden fat in Indian
foods. Here are just a few figures for popular items to warn you
to steer clear of them in general, although some fibre-rich dhals
could be included in your menus.

BOMBAY POTATO, per 300g
   portion ....................................**5**
CANNED LENTIL DHAL, half a
   400g can ................................**3**
CANNED CHICK PEA DHAL,
   half a 400g can ......................**2**
CHICKEN TIKKA MASALA,
   per 300g portion ..................**11**
CHICKEN TANDOORI, per
   175g portion........................**6½**
CURRY PASTE per 15ml/
   1 level tablespoon ..................**2**
CURRY PASTE, slightly
   rounded teaspoon ..................**1**
CURRY POWDER .................**0**

GOBI ALOO SAAG, per 300g
   portion .................................**8½**
LAMB KHEEMA, per 300g
   portion....................................**14**
LAMB ROGAN JOSH, per
   300g portion ..........................**9**
ONION BHAJI, 50g .............**2½**
VEGETABLE SAMOSA, 50g**2½**

## INDIAN MEAL ACCOMPANIMENTS
CHAPATTI, per 50g portion ....**2**
NAAN BREAD, per 50g
   portion ................................**1½**
PAPPADUM, each .................**1**

# ● MAYONNAISE (AND MAYONNAISE-BASED SAUCES)

If foods were rated for their figure-threat factors mayonnaise might well top the list. Chocolate you *know* is fattening! Mayonnaise, lavishly used these days in so many foods, is a far more secret and therefore sinister threat. It can, and does, turn most ready-made sandwiches and coleslaw into very fattening foods. Even reduced-fat and light mayonnaises, a much better choice, contain a significant quantity of fatty calories.

You have been warned. Hold the mayonnaise. Or at least go for the light reduced-fat varieties, which are no real sacrifice, and measure them carefully. Here we've given fat units per 15ml tablespoon – a *level* tablespoon! – for mayonnaise-based sauces such as the ubiquitous tartare sauce, as well as mayonnaise itself.

MAYONNAISE, per level
    tablespoon ..............................**4**
MAYONNAISE, REDUCED-
    FAT OR LIGHT, per level
    tablespoon ..........................**1½**
MAYONNAISE, EXTRA LIGHT,
    per tablespoon ......................**½**

## MAYONNAISE-BASED SAUCES

CORONATION SAUCE, per
    level tablespoon ..................**1½**
TARTARE SAUCE, per level
    tablespoon ..........................**1½**
SEAFOOD SAUCE, per level
    tablespoon ............................ **2**
REDUCED-FAT SEAFOOD
    SAUCE, per level tablespoon **1**

See page 155 for other salad dressings.

# ● MEAT

The excess of red and processed meat (such as bacon, sausages, salamis and other deli products) in typical Western diets has been linked in many recent scientific studies to major diseases. Even lean meat. Check back to pages 31–2 to see what's going on in your colon after you've eaten meat and why we advise you to limit it to no more than two helpings a week.

Lower the meat content and boost the vegetable content of popular dishes such as cottage pie with the recipes in this book. And give Quorn products a try as low-fat meat-free alternatives to popular meat dishes.

**All fat units are given per 25g/1oz unless otherwise stated.**

## BACON AND HAM

BACON, per rasher, back or
streaky, grilled ....................**1½**

GAMMON, average steak (250g/
9oz raw weight) grilled ........**5½**

HAM, cooked weight, lean
only ..........................................**½**

HAM, cooked weight, lean
and fat .................................**1½**

## BEEF

CORNED BEEF ......................**1**

ROAST BEEF, lean only ..........**1**

ROAST BEEF, lean and fat ..**1½**

LEAN GRILLING STEAK,
average, weighed raw............**½**

SMALL (175g/6oz raw weight)
lean steak, grilled, each..........**3**

AVERAGE SIZED (225g/8oz
raw weight) lean steak, grilled,
each .........................................**4**

MINCED BEEF, weighed
raw .......................................**1½**

LEAN MINCED BEEF (less
than 10% fat), weighed raw ..**1**

## BURGERS

Although different brands vary a little in fat content, the following figures will be close enough to keep fat and calorie intake at weight-loss level.

**Fat units are given for whole grilled burger in each case.**

SMALL BURGER, 50g/2oz raw
weight .....................................**3**

LARGE BURGER, 115g/4oz
raw weight .............................**7**

## LAMB

LEG, roasted, lean only ............**1**

LEG, roasted, lean and fat ....**1½**

SHOULDER, roasted, lean and
fat............................................**2**

AVERAGE CHUMP CHOP
(150g/5oz raw weight),
grilled .......................................**8**

AVERAGE LOIN CHOP (125g/
4½oz raw weight) grilled..........**7**

## LIVER

CHICKEN LIVER, per 50g/2oz
raw ..........................................**½**

LAMB'S LIVER, fried............**1½**

LAMB'S LIVER, raw ..............**½**

LIVER PÂTÉ ........................**3½**

143

LIVER PÂTÉ, reduced-fat ......½

## PORK

FILLET, lean only, raw ............½
LEG JOINT, roasted, lean and
fat..............................................**1**
LOIN CHOP, 125g/4½oz raw
weight, grilled ........................**4**
PORK CHOP, 200g/7oz raw
weight, grilled ......................**6½**

## SAUSAGES

Fat units are given per whole
sausage, well grilled to drain
off maximum fat. See Quorn
section for lower-fat alternatives.

BEEF SAUSAGE, large ..........**3**
BEEF SAUSAGE, thin..........**1½**
PORK SAUSAGE, large ......**3½**
PORK SAUSAGE, thin ............**2**

## ● MEXICAN FOODS

Mexican foods give maximum flavour kick for calories to spice
up your diet. We were cheered to find that even refried beans
aren't as fatty as they sound when we checked out Old El Paso
and Discovery, the leading supermarket brands.

FAJITA SPICE MIX, per 35g
sachet .....................................½
REFRIED BEANS, per 215g
can ...........................................½
SALSA, CHILLED, per average
170g pot ................................**1**
SOURED CREAM, fresh or
long-life, per *level* tablespoon **1**
TACO SHELLS, EACH............**1**
TORTILLAS, CORN, EACH....**1**
TORTILLAS, WHEAT FLOUR,
EACH......................................**1**

## SAUCES, PER JAR AS SOLD:

DISCOVERY CHILLI CON
CARNE SAUCE, 370g ......**1½**
DISCOVERY FAJITA SAUCE,
370g ....................................**3½**
OLD EL PASO ENCHILADA
SAUCE, 475g.....................**6½**
OLD EL PASO FAJITA SAUCE,
475g.......................................**1**
OLD EL PASO SIZZLING
SAUCE, 235g .......................**4**
UNCLE BEN'S CHILLI CON
CARNE SAUCE, 500g ..........**1**

# ● MILK

We suggest skimmed organic dairy or calcium-enriched unsweetened soya as the best milks to use in cereals and tea, for reasons explained on page 97. Here are the fat units to count if you do – and the extras to add, which come mainly in the form of that unhealthy saturated fat, if you don't. Some recent studies suggest that the milk from organically reared cows is a better source of important nutrients than that of non-organic cows, because they eat more fresh grass and clover and a generally more natural diet.

**Units are given for half a pint (300ml) in each case.**

## RECOMMENDED MILKS

SKIMMED DAIRY MILK ........½
UNSWEETENED SOYA
   MILK ...................................1½

## OTHER MILKS

COW'S BREAKFAST MILK....5
COW'S CHANNEL ISLAND
   MILK ...................................5½
COW'S FULL-FAT MILK ........4
COW'S SEMI-SKIMMED
   MILK ........................................2
GOAT'S MILK ..........................4

# ● MUFFINS

You see them here, you see them there, these days you see them everywhere. But take a look at these typical fat figures before you thank the USA for this particular blessing. One thing in their favour is that muffins are usually bought singly rather than in packs. But here we're clearly talking in terms of only an occasional – *very* occasional – treat.

LARGE BLUEBERRY MUFFIN
   (approx 120g)..........................8
MEDIUM-SIZED BLUEBERRY
   MUFFIN...................................5
MINI BLUEBERRY MUFFIN
   (SOLD IN MULTI-PACKS)....2
LARGE DOUBLE
   CHOCOLATE CHIP
   MUFFIN (approx 120g) ......9½

MEDIUM-SIZED DOUBLE
   CHOCOLATE CHIP
   MUFFIN ...............................6
MINI DOUBLE CHOCOLATE
   CHIP MUFFIN (SOLD IN
   MULTI-PACKS) .................2½

# ● **NUTS**

Although cram-packed with valuable nutrients, nuts are also cram-packed with calorie-rich oil. And it's just so easy to eat lots of them in a very short time – so hard to stop once you've opened a packet. Eaten with alcohol, as they so often are, nuts pose an even greater hazard for slimmers. The nuts make you want more alcohol, the alcohol makes you want more nuts . . .

## Advice for dieters:
- Don't eat nuts with an alcoholic drink.
- Only ever buy the smallest individual-sized packet.
- Ideally choose pistachio nuts, sold in their shells. Having to shell each one slows down eating speed considerably and makes you content with less.

## Health note
When eaten salted, nuts can add to excess salt intake. Salt won't affect your weight but is linked with high blood pressure and strokes.

**Fat units are given per 25g/1oz, weighed shelled unless otherwise stated.**

ALMONDS ............................**5½**

ALMONDS, blanched, whole or flaked ....................................**5½**

ONE WHOLE ALMOND ........**½**

MARZIPAN ..........................**1½**

BRAZIL NUTS ......................**7**

ONE WHOLE BRAZIL NUT ....................................**1**

CASHEW NUTS ....................**5**

CHESTNUTS, weighed shelled ....................................**1**

COCONUT, creamed block......**7**

COCONUT, desiccated............**6**

COCONUT MILK, per 400ml can....................................**24**

COCONUT MILK, REDUCED FAT, per 400ml can ..............**12**

COCONUT CREAM, per 200ml carton ..................................**16**

HAZELNUTS ........................**6½**

MACADAMIA NUTS ..............**8**

MIXED NUTS AND RAISINS..............................**3½**

PEANUTS, DRY ROASTED..............................**5**

PEANUTS, ROASTED SALTED ............................**5½**

PEANUT BUTTER, per teaspoon............................**1½**

PECANS ................................**7**

PINE NUTS ..............................**7**

PISTACHIO NUTS, weighed
with shells ...........................**3**

PISTACHIO NUTS, weighed
shelled ..............................**5½**

WALNUTS...............................**7**

## ● OILS

Whether olive, corn, palm, safflower, sesame, soya, sunflower, peanut, walnut – you name it – oil is oil in terms of the whopping number of fatty calories it supplies. Ration it strictly. Measure it carefully. Every drop counts when you are trying to lose weight. Sorry to nag, but don't live another day without owning measuring spoons. You'll find these in kitchenware departments.

When rationing fats for weight loss it's particularly important to focus on healthier oils in place of solid saturated and trans fats. Read about them on pages 124–7.

**ALL OILS**
Per 15ml tablespoon ..............**5**
Per 5ml teaspoon ..................**2**

## ● PASTA SAUCES

Forget (*please!*) that totally misleading low-carb nonsense about pasta being fattening. It's the sauce that makes the real differ-ence to a pasta meal. Choose the right one and wholewheat pasta, with a side salad, is among the most healthy and helpful of all dieting meals: high fibre, low GI, low cal, filling, easy. Choose the wrong one and you're downing loads of fatty calo-ries. You get a main-course portion of pasta (90–100g dry weight) for around 300 calories – well within weight-loss limits for a main meal – but could more than double this by adding an oily sauce. In cheesy sauces many calories will be in the form of health-threatening saturated fat.

You'll find recipes for low-fat pasta sauces on pages 168–70 and some answers to 'Heavens, I haven't got time – what can I eat tonight?' emergencies below.

the fat and calorie controller

We've trawled the stores to select some of the lowest-fat ready-made pasta sauces. We also give figures for some of the worst to show just how picky you have to be.

## CHILLED CARTON SAUCES

Supermarkets' own brands don't vary significantly in fat content. Safest chilled sauces are Napoletana, Arrabbiata and Amatriciana. The most figure-threatening are those containing cheese.

**Fat units per 350g pot:**

| | |
|---|---|
| AMATRICIANA .........................**3** | REDUCED-FAT |
| ARRABBIATA.......................**2½** |   CARBONARA.......................**5** |
| CARBONARA.......................**17** | REDUCED-FAT CHEESE ....**4½** |
| CHEESE .................................**15** | TOMATO AND |
| NAPOLETANA.....................**3½** |   MASCARPONE ..................**10** |

## LOW-FAT JARS AND POUCHES

Some of the lowest-fat sauces are in jars and pouches in the Dolmio and Ragu range. Sacla and Seeds of Change also include some reasonable low-fat choices.

### DOLMIO

**Fat units per 320 jar:**

BOLOGNESE LIGHT..............**½**

EXTRA MUSHROOM
  BOLOGNAISE ......................**1**

EXTRA SPICY BOLOGNAISE**1**

ORIGINAL BOLOGNAISE ..**1½**

### DOLMIO EXPRESS

**Fat units per 170g pouch:**

BOLOGNESE ..........................**2**

CREAMY CARBONARA .......**8**

EXTRA MUSHROOM
  BOLOGNESE ......................**2**

EXTRA ONION AND GARLIC

BOLOGNESE ..........................**2**

RICH TOMATO, BASIL AND
  PESTO ...............................**3½**

SPICY ITALIAN CHILLI .........**1**

TOMATO AND BASIL ...........**1**

### RAGU

**Fat units per 275g jar:**

RAGU TRADITIONAL..........**1½**

### SACLA

**Fat units per 290g jar:**

WHOLE CHERRY TOMATO
  AND BASIL............................**5**

WHOLE CHERRY TOMATO
  AND CHILLI ......................**1½**

## SEEDS OF CHANGE ORGANIC

**Fat units per 350g jar:**

CHERRY TOMATO AND
OLIVE .....................................4

CHILLI JALAPENO
PEPPER.............................8½

MEDITERRANEAN
VEGETABLE .........................4

## CHOOSE WITH CARE FROM THESE!

As long as you use just half a jar or less, some products in the Loyd Grossman and Napolina ranges could squeeze into your diet. Others, though, are very rich in oil. There are a full 14½ fat units in a full jar of Napolina Carbonara, for example. We've picked out some of the least oily in these ranges.

## LOYD GROSSMAN

**Per 350g jar:**

BOLOGNESE .......................3½
SWEET RED PEPPER............7
TOMATO AND CHARGRILLED
VEGETABLES.......................7
TOMATO AND CHILLI ...........7
TOMATO & WILD
MUSHROOM ........................7

## NAPOLINA

**Per 325g jar:**

TOMATO, CHILLI AND
GARLIC ..............................6½
TOMATO AND MIXED
PEPPERS .........................5½

## THE DODGY LOT

In general, steer clear of 'Stir Through' and 'Stir In' sauces in any range. These contain a particularly high proportion of oil to coat the pasta. We give some examples below, plus one low-fat version. Pesto, the original stir-in sauce, is universally high – *very* high – in fat, whatever the make. If you only use a little (as you might with some of these sauces), make sure it is a carefully measured 'little'.

## PESTO

**Note that fat units are given for just 25g/1oz:**

GREEN PESTO ....................4½
RED PESTO ........................3½

## SACLA STIR-THROUGH SAUCES

**Per 190g pot:**

OLIVE AND TOMATO ..........12
SPICY PEPPER AND
TOMATO ................................8

the fat and calorie controller

SUN-DRIED TOMATO AND
  GARLIC ....................................**9**
VINE-RIPENED TOMATO AND
  MASCARPONE .............**10½**

## DOLMIO STIR-IN SAUCE

**Per 150g pot of this lower-fat choice:**
SUN-DRIED TOMATO
  LIGHT ..............................**2½**

## ● PASTRY

Don't even go there! All pastry products are very fattening and
rarely something you really *crave*. Be strong. Resist. You can.
These figures will help to stiffen your back-bone.

### DANISH PASTRIES
**Per average pastry,**
  100g/3½oz ............................**6**

### PASTIES
**Per pasty:**
CHEESE AND ONION PASTY,
  150g/5oz .............................**9½**
CORNISH PASTY, 225g/
  8oz ...................................**14½**

### PASTRY ROLLS
**Per roll:**
CHEESE AND ONION ROLL,
  medium, 70g/2½oz .................**5**
SAUSAGE ROLL, MINI, 35g/
  1¼oz ....................................**3½**

SAUSAGE ROLL, MEDIUM,
  70g/2½oz ..............................**7**
SAUSAGE ROLL, LARGE,
  100g/3½oz ...........................**10**

### PORK PIES
**Per pie:**
MINI, 50g/2oz ......................**4½**
SNACK SIZE, 75g/3oz ............**8**
INDIVIDUAL PORK PIE,
  140g/4¾oz ...........................**12**

### QUICHE
**Per 115g/4oz slice:**
CHEESE AND ONION
  QUICHE ...............................**9**
QUICHE LORRAINE .............**9**

## ● PÂTÉ

Very fatty stuff, pâté. If you eat any at all, choose only those
labelled 'reduced fat'. Remember the processed-meat health
rule: 'No more than twice a week'.

**Fat units per 25g/1oz:**

ARDENNE .................................3
ARDENNE, REDUCED
  FAT ......................................1½
BRUSSELS ..........................3½

BRUSSELS, REDUCED
  FAT .......................................1½
CHICKEN LIVER .................3½
DUCK AND ORANGE ............3

## ● PIZZAS

Pizzas can range from the 'permissible' to the 'terminal' where weight is concerned. It isn't the base, it's all those fatty, cheesy calories – even worse, fatty cheesy and meaty calories! – heaped on top that makes the difference. Thick bottom, thin top is a good rule of thumb to get maximum filling power for minimum fattening power. There's little advantage in a thin base but the less cheese and meat on top the better. And always serve pizza with a pulse-packed F2 Salads to add that essential fibre and lower the GI of the meal.

### You can limit fatty pizza calories by:
- Buying a pizza base and topping it yourself.
- Choosing pizzas labelled 'low fat', available in most super-markets, or the small frozen French bread type.
- Choosing a mini-sized pizza and eating it with loads of salad.

Pizza-eaters should brace themselves for some shock-horror figures below. And you wondered why you were putting on weight? Nearly every restaurant pizza, unless there's a cheese-free option, costs around 1,000 calories. By far the most lethal of the shop-bought lot are those labelled 'stuffed crust' (cheese inside as well as on top), 'loaded cheese', 'meat feast' and 'deep pan'. As many as 1,300 calories and enough fat to give a bullock a heart attack in one of those.

## PUT-IT-TOGETHER PIZZA INGREDIENTS:

NAPOLINA MINI PIZZA BASE
(14cm/5½ inch) per base ........**1**

NAPOLINA LARGE PIZZA
BASE (23cm/9 inch)
per base ..............................**1½**

NAPOLINA PIZZA TOPPING,
per 300g jar ........................**2½**

## REDUCED-FAT PIZZAS

REDUCED-FAT CHEESE AND
TOMATO PIZZA (18cm/
7 inch)..................................**2½**

REDUCED-FAT HAM AND
PINEAPPLE PIZZA (18cm/
7 inch) ....................................**3**

REDUCED-FAT ROASTED
VEGETABLE (18cm/7 inch)....**3**

## SMALL PIZZAS

AVERAGE CHEESE AND
TOMATO PIZZA (13cm/
5 inch) ....................................**2**

CHICAGO DEEP DISH
FROZEN MINI PIZZAS (2 in
a pack)

HAM AND PINEAPPLE, per
mini pizza ...........................**5½**

HOT AND SPICY, per mini
pizza ...................................**6½**

TRIPLE CHEESE, per mini
pizza......................................**4**

PIZZA FINGERS (10 in a frozen
pack) per pizza finger ............**½**

FRENCH BREAD PIZZAS
FINDUS FRENCH BREAD
CHEESE AND TOMATO
PIZZA, each ..........................**1**

## SHOCK-HORROR PIZZAS!

DEEP-LOADED CHEESE
PIZZA (25cm/10 inch) per
pizza..................................**17½**

DEEP-PAN PEPPERONI
PIZZA (20cm/8 inch) per
pizza..................................**18½**

STUFFED-CRUST MEAT
FEAST PIZZA (25cm/10 inch)
per pizza .............................**18**

## ● POULTRY

### CHICKEN

Lean skinless chicken can be a low-fat food if you opt for free-
range – ideally organic free-range. Recent research suggests
that factory-farmed chicken (which means all chicken on sale

not labelled 'free-range' or 'organic') now has a higher fat content than was previously realized, thanks to so-called 'advances' in the speed of chicken growth. Avoid fast-food fried chicken and fat-added ready-made chicken meals which can be very high in fat content and calories, as you can see from the figures below. Fat units given for basic chicken meat apply to free-range and free-range organic.

**All fat units are given per 25g/1oz unless otherwise stated.**

BREAST MEAT, roasted, eaten without skin..............................½

LEG MEAT, roasted, eaten without skin ............................1

AVERAGE BREAST, eaten without skin, cooked without fat ..........................................½

DRUMSTICKS, roasted or grilled with skin, each..........1½

LEG QUARTER, roasted or barbecued, eaten with skin **7½**

## POPULAR CHICKEN DISHES

CHICKEN NUGGETS (6) ........**5**

CHICKEN TIKKA MASALA, per 300g portion...................**11**

CHICKEN KIEV, per 150g portion....................................**12**

## TAKE-AWAY FRIED COATED CHICKEN

**Per piece:**

CRISPY STRIP ........................**2**

DRUMSTICK............................**4**

THIGH .......................................**7**

WING ....................................**4½**

## DUCK

**Per 25g/1oz unless otherwise stated.**

DUCK, CRISPY, Chinese style ......................................**2½**

DUCK, ROAST, lean meat only ...........................................**1**

DUCK, ROAST, lean and fat with skin...................................**4**

DUCK, BREAST FILLET, per 175g/6oz raw breast, grilled or baked, eaten with skin ........**10**

DUCK, BREAST FILLET, per 175g/6oz raw breast, grilled or baked, eaten without skin............................................**3**

## TURKEY

BREAST MEAT, roasted, eaten without skin..............................½

# ● QUORN FOODS

Quorn alternatives to meat, once only eaten by vegetarians, have gained widespread popularity since so many people with cholesterol problems have been given doctor's orders to 'cut that saturated fat'. Most contain fewer calories than equivalent meat products. You'll find Quorn products prominently displayed in the chilled-food departments of supermarkets.

**Fat units are given for items as sold or cooked without fat unless otherwise stated.**

QUORN BURGERS, per burger.................................**1**

QUORN SOUTHERN STYLE BURGERS, per burger ..........**2**

QUORN SAUSAGES, per sausage.....................................½

QUORN SLICES, HAM FLAVOUR, per 50g/2oz ........½

QUORN SLICES, TURKEY FLAVOUR with stuffing, per 25g/1oz ....................................½

QUORN COTTAGE PIE, per whole pack ..........................**2½**

QUORN FILLET......................½

QUORN GARLIC AND HERB FILLET ..............................**1½**

QUORN LEMON AND BLACK PEPPER FILLET ..................**3**

QUORN PORK STYLE RIBSTER, 2 ribsters..............½

QUORN MINCE OR PIECES, per 50g/2oz............................½

QUORN SOUTHERN STYLE NUGGETS, per nugget ........½

# ● RATATOUILLE

This lovely mix of veg in its own sauce can make a meal in itself, served with, for instance, green beans, mushrooms and maybe a baked potato. See recipe on page 201.

**For shop-bought next-best versions, fat units are counted below.**

PER 400g CAN RATATOUILLE ......................**3**

PER 300g CHILLED CARTON RATATOUILLE ......................**2**

# ● SALAD DRESSINGS

Take care – like mayonnaise, most salad dressings are very high in calories. Options for slimmers include making your own with a lower ratio of oil to vinegar, trying low-fat or fat-free shop-bought dressings, or having just a small quantity of the one you love best. Either way, measure it carefully and count the fat units.

**Fat units are given per 15ml tablespoon unless otherwise stated.**

BALSAMIC VINEGAR
  DRESSING, shop bought......**3**
BLUE CHEESE DRESSING,
  shop bought ........................**2½**
CAESAR DRESSING, shop
  bought ....................................**3**
CAESAR DRESSING, LOW
  FAT, 2 tbsp ............................**½**
FRENCH (VINAIGRETTE)
  DRESSING, shop bought ....**3**
FRENCH (VINAIGRETTE)
  DRESSING, REDUCED FAT,
  shop bought, 2tbsp ..............**½**
FRENCH (VINAIGRETTE)
  DRESSING, FAT FREE, shop
  bought ....................................**0**
FRENCH (VINAIGRETTE)
  DRESSING, HOMEMADE
  (3 tbsp oil to 1 tbsp vinegar) ..**4**
FRENCH (VINAIGRETTE)
  DRESSING, HOMEMADE
  (2 tbsp oil to 1tbsp vinegar) **3½**

HERB AND GARLIC
  DRESSING, shop bought......**2**
HERB AND GARLIC
  DRESSING, shop bought, low
  fat ............................................**½**
HONEY AND MUSTARD
  DRESSING, shop bought......**2**
HONEY AND MUSTARD
  DRESSING, low fat...............**1**
ITALIAN DRESSING, shop
  bought ....................................**3**
ITALIAN DRESSING, shop
  bought, low fat, 2 tbsp ..........**½**
SALAD CREAM....................**1½**
SALAD CREAM, light or
  reduced fat.............................**1**
THOUSAND ISLAND, shop
  bought ..................................**1½**
THOUSAND ISLAND, shop
  bought, reduced fat................**1**

# ● SEEDS

Suddenly seeds are sexy – and for sound reasons, on the whole. Some, in particular flaxseeds (linseeds) and hemp seeds, help supply Omega 3 fatty acids, the only fat-based nutrients we are likely to lack. Like nuts, seeds are high in fatty calories, but lack their 'once you start you can't stop' factor. No woman (at least to our knowledge) has grown fat due to an irresistible urge to binge on seeds. But if you choose to include them in your diet for health benefits, their fat content certainly needs to be taken into account.

**Fat units are given per 25g/1oz.**

| | | | |
|---|---|---|---|
| FLAX SEEDS | 4½ | SESAME SEEDS | 5½ |
| HEMP SEEDS | 3 | SUNFLOWER SEEDS | 5 |
| LINSEEDS | 4½ | TAHINI PASTE (used in | |
| POPPY SEEDS | 4½ | houmous), per teaspoon | 1 |

# ● SHELLFISH AND SEAFOOD

Although seafood is a source of dietary cholesterol (the cholesterol you eat, as opposed to the cholesterol your own body makes), F2 strictly rations saturated fats, which are the major cause of cholesterol problems. So most people – check with your doctor if you have heart health problems – can afford to enjoy a little seafood in their diet. As you see, it is low in fatty calories.

**Fat units are given per 25g/1oz unless otherwise stated.**

| | | | |
|---|---|---|---|
| CALAMARI, FRIED IN BATTER | 1 | PRAWNS, peeled, per 75g/3oz portion | ½ |
| CALAMARI, RAW, per 75g/3oz | ½ | SCALLOPS, raw, per 75g/3oz | ½ |
| CRAB MEAT, light and dark meat | ½ | SCAMPI IN BREADCRUMBS, frozen | 1 |
| LOBSTER, per 115g/4oz portion | ½ | SCAMPI IN BREADCRUMBS, deep fried | 1½ |
| MUSSELS, SHELLED | ½ | SEAFOOD STICKS, per 115g/4oz portion | ½ |
| MUSSELS, weighed with shells, per 115g/4oz | ½ | SEAFOOD SELECTION, per 75g/3oz portion | ½ |

## ● STIR-FRY SAUCES

Mounds of veg, quick-fried in hardly any oil, make a stir-fry a very virtuous F2 meal. Use a good non-stick pan and discover how very little oil you need.

Suffer no guilt if you save time by using ready-prepared stir-fry veg packs, but take care if choosing ready-made stir-fry sauces. These vary vastly in fat content. You can make your own with the recipes on page 196 or choose the low-fat varieties from the leading brands listed below. We've included a few high-fat sauces just to emphasize how very choosy you have to be. Many of these sachets contain more than is necessary for a single stir-fry meal. Don't use any more than you need.

Oyster, Soy and Nam Pla Thai fish sauces are virtually fat-free, but go easy on them for health because they are all salty.

### AMOY

**Per 150g sachet:**

AROMATIC BLACK BEAN ....½
CLASSIC SWEET AND
  SOUR .....................................½
CRACKED BLACK
  PEPPER.............................2½
PERFECT PLUM .....................½
ROASTED PEANUT SATAY 9½
RICH OYSTER AND GARLIC ½
SWEET SOY CHOW MEIN ....3

### BLUE DRAGON

**Per 120g sachet:**

CANTON BLACK BEAN ........1
CHOP SUEY ...........................1
CHOW MEIN...........................1
HOISIN AND GARLIC..........1½
OYSTER AND SPRING
  ONION ..................................½
PEKING LEMON .....................1
SWEET AND SOUR ..............½

SZECHUAN SPICY
  TOMATO ...........................2½
TERIYAKI .............................½
THAI GREEN CURRY..........1½
THAI NOODLE ........................2

### KEN HOM

**Per jar:**

BLACK BEAN WITH ORANGE
  AND LIME, 210g ................3½
CHILLI AND GARLIC WITH
  JALAPENO PEPPERS,
  220g .....................................½
SWEET AND SOUR WITH
  PASSION FRUIT, 220g ........½
THAI GREEN CURRY WITH
  LEMON GRASS, 200g ......9½

### SHARWOODS

**Per 195g jar:**

BLACK BEAN ....................10½
HOISIN .....................................½
LEMON AND SESAME..........½

SPICY TOMATO
SZECHUAN ..........................½
SWEET CHILLI AND LEMON
GRASS ..................................½

SWEET AND SOUR ..............½
TERIYAKI BLACK PEPPER ..½
YELLOW BEAN ......................½

## ● SUSHI

Before their 'conversion' by McMissionaries, the Japanese boasted some of the world's slimmest waistlines and a life expectancy of eighty-plus on their traditional diet of vegetables, rice and fish. Now their waistlines have expanded and life expectancy has contracted as many follow a Westernized diet. The good news is the growing popularity of traditional Japanese food in the West. Sushi selections vary from pack to pack and restaurant to restaurant, but this is basically low-fat food and you can safely estimate the following units.

**Per average 150g pack:**
FISH SUSHI..........................**1½**
VEGETABLE SUSHI ............**1½**

## ● YOGURTS

One low-fat probiotic drink or yogurt daily, to supplement the good bacteria in your body, is part of F2's formula, but from time to time you might also want to use other yogurts in place of cream or for snacks or puds. Here are the fat units to count:

### BEST CHOICES
ALPRO SOYA FRUIT
YOGURTS, per 125g pot ......**1**
FRUIT OR NATURAL LOW-
FAT DAIRY YOGURTS, per
150g pot ................................**½**

### OTHER YOGURTS
FRUIT OR NATURAL YOGURT,
whole milk, per 150g pot ....**1½**

GREEK-STYLE YOGURT,
cow's milk, natural, per 100g/
3½oz .....................................**3½**
GREEK-STYLE YOGURT,
cow's milk, natural, per level
tablespoon ............................**½**
GREEK-STYLE YOGURT,
sheep's milk, natural, per
100g/3½oz ..............................**2**

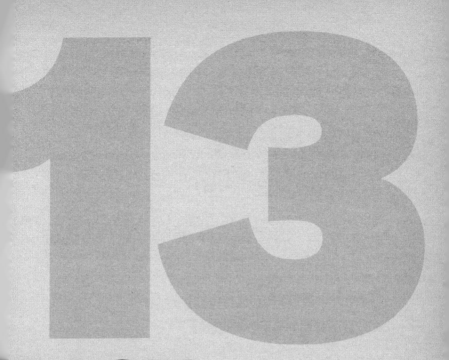

# 13
# EASY
# MEALS

ANYONE WHO imagines dieters can turn to recipes for every meal hasn't tried to diet or doesn't have a life. Sometimes – often – you only have time to fix something really simple. Here, without apologies, is a selection of easy, effortless and sometimes obvious meals which fit in with the **F2** health and weight-loss formula. We've counted them for fat units for you. Turn to this section when you are pressed for time or can't think what to eat.

# Something simple on wholemeal toast

Most of these toast-toppings are moist enough to eliminate the need for fatty spreads, and in some instances we've suggested alternative spreads. Serve these on your two daily slices of wholemeal bread, toasted, or on one slice after a bowl of **F2** Soup or with **F2** Salads.

## On two slices of toast:

### Poached eggs

Lightly poach two Omega-3 free-range, medium-sized eggs. Serve on two slices of hot toast. If liked, first spread the toast with a little mustard, Marmite, or (at the cost of another ½ fat unit) olive tapenade.

## Good old baked beans

Spread two slices of toast thinly with brown sauce, if liked, then top with a can of heated-up baked beans.

## Chilli beans

Heat half a 400g can of red kidney or mixed beans which have been canned in a spicy or chilli sauce. Mix in some finely chopped onion and chopped peppers or sweetcorn – or both. Pile on two slices of hot toast.

## Pizza style

Grill two thickly sliced tomatoes on foil in a grill pan with some crushed garlic and a sprinkling of dried mixed herbs or seasoning. Spread two slices of hot toast with a little tomato purée and top with the tomatoes. Scatter with four drained anchovies, a few sliced black olives and capers. Serve with a ready-made **F2** Salad.

## Spiced banana and honey

Mash one large banana with 1–2 tsp honey, to taste, a few sultanas and a pinch of ground cinnamon. Spread on two slices of hot toast.

# On one slice of toast, with soup or salad:

## Sardines with pesto

Spread one slice of hot toast thinly with 1 teaspoon pesto sauce, lay sliced tomatoes on top. Mash two well-drained sardines, the kind which have been canned in brine, with a splash of vinegar to liven the flavour (and lower the GI), and spread on top of the tomatoes.

### Sardines and cucumber

Mash two sardines canned in tomato sauce with some of the sauce and a splash of vinegar. Spread on one slice of hot toast then top with sliced cucumber. Serve with cherry tomatoes and a ready-made **F2** Salad.

### Cheese and celery

Spread one slice of lightly browned toast with 50g/2oz light (half-fat) soft cheese with chives, mixed with one stick finely chopped celery. Pop under a preheated grill to warm through. Serve with cherry tomatoes, a ready-made **F2** Salad and Branston or another favourite pickle if liked.

# A sandwich, soup and fruit

Most shop-bought sandwiches are high in fatty calories. Make your own healthy **F2** versions, using fibre-rich wholemeal bread. If you lunch at home, or can heat soup at the office (or take a flask), one sandwich with a bowl of ready-made **F2** soup would make an ideal midday meal. Follow it with a piece of fruit from our high-fi selection on page 91 and your good bacteria will feast all afternoon.

Here are some simple ideas for sandwich fillings. We've cut back on the usual lavish quantities of mayonnaise, used only the light lower-calorie type and suggested spreads other than butter or margarine. In some cases the sandwiches will be best if you pack filling and bread separately and assemble them at lunchtime. These days many offices have fridges in which fillings could be stored.

Quantities are given for filling one sandwich made from your daily two large slices of wholemeal bread.

---

# NOTE OF CAUTION

All spoon measurements are level and proper measuring spoons are essential – particularly for mayonnaise. Use the light (reduced-fat) mayonnaise, 1½ fat units per tbsp, rather than regular full-fat mayonnaise at a whopping 4 fat units per tbsp. All units below have been calculated using light mayonnaise. To further reduce fat you could opt for extra-light mayonnaise at only ½ fat unit per tbsp.

---

## Houmous and tomato or roasted pepper

**FAT UNITS 3**

Spread bread with up to 50g/2oz (3 tbsp) reduced-fat houmous. Fill sandwich with sliced tomato or a sliced roasted red pepper and a handful of rocket leaves. You can buy roasted red peppers packed in vinegar in jars or from a deli counter. Drain them thoroughly.

## Spicy prawn

**FAT UNITS 4**

Stir 1tsp of mango chutney and ½tsp mild curry paste into 2 tbsp light, reduced-fat mayonnaise. Spread a little of this mixture on each slice of bread. Squeeze just a little lemon juice on 2–3 oz prawns and stir in the remaining mayonnaise. Fill sandwich with prawn mayonnaise, crunchy lettuce leaves and cucumber.

## Tuna and sweetcorn

Blend 2 tbsp light mayonnaise with 50g/2oz drained tuna (canned in brine or spring water), 1 tbsp sweetcorn and a few capers. Spread between slices of bread and pack out with shredded lettuce. No spread needed on the bread.

## Tuna and bean

Combine 2 tbsp light mayonnaise with 1tsp tomato purée or ketchup. Spread a little of this mixture on each slice of bread. Stir 50g/2oz drained tuna (canned in brine or spring water), 1tbsp drained, canned red kidney beans and some finely chopped red onion into the remaining mayonnaise. Spread between the bread.

## Peanut butter and banana

Spread each slice of bread with 1tsp smooth or crunchy peanut butter (2 tsp in total). Fill sandwich with mashed or sliced banana.

## Peanut butter with crunchy salad

Spread each slice of bread with 1tsp crunchy peanut butter (2 tsp in total). Fill with sliced cucumber and a handful of raw bean sprouts. Sprinkle with a little sweet chilli sauce for a spicy Thai-style flavour, if you like.

## Mashed banana with walnuts

Mash 1 large banana with 1–2 tsp honey and 15g/½oz chopped walnuts. Spread between slices of bread. No spread is needed on the bread.

## Cottage cheese and Marmite

Spread 1 slice of bread with 1tsp low-fat spread and the other slice thinly with Marmite. Fill sandwich with 50g/2oz plain cottage cheese, drained, sliced cucumber and shredded lettuce.

## Turkey and cranberry

Spread bread with 1tbsp cranberry sauce, then fill sandwich with 50g/2oz thinly sliced, skinless, free-range or organic roast turkey or chicken breast.

## Smoked salmon and soft cheese

Spread bread with 50g/2oz (3 tbsp) half-fat soft cheese, flavoured with snipped chives or a few chopped capers if liked. Fill with 25g/1oz thinly sliced organic smoked salmon, sprinkled with black pepper and a little lemon juice. Pack out with baby spinach leaves or watercress.

## Canned salmon and watercress

Blend 2 tbsp light mayonnaise with the grated zest of ½ lemon and 1tsp lemon juice. Spread a little of the mayonnaise on the bread. Stir 50g/2oz drained canned pink salmon (wild Pacific) into the remaining mayonnaise for the filling and pack out with trimmed watercress.

## Egg, watercress and tomato

Mash one medium hard-boiled egg (free-range, Omega 3) with 1tbsp light mayonnaise and some chopped watercress. Scoop the seeds out of one largish tomato, dice the remaining flesh and add to the egg.

Season and spread between the slices of bread. No spread is needed on the bread.

## Cheese, carrot and sultana

Mature cheddar cheese – more flavour for your calories – makes the best **F2** cheese choice and this sandwich filling makes a little go a long way. Grate 25g/1oz and combine with a small grated carrot, 1tbsp sultanas and 1tsp light mayonnaise. Blend together an additional teaspoon of light mayonnaise with one of wholegrain mustard and spread on the bread. Fill the sandwich with the cheese and carrot mixture.

## Crab with sweetcorn

Mix 100g/3½oz drained white canned crabmeat with 2tbsp sweetcorn, 2 tbsp light mayonnaise and 1tsp tomato ketchup. Spice with a dash of Tabasco sauce. Sandwich between slices of bread. No spread is needed on the bread.

## Chicken with pineapple and almonds

Mix 50g/2oz diced cooked organic chicken with 2 tbsp light mayonnaise. Stir in a chopped ring of canned pineapple, drained of juice, ¼ of a green pepper, diced, and 5g (about 10 flakes) of toasted almonds. Don't be tempted to add extra almonds as they are high in fat, but, toasted, they add a lovely flavour to this filling. Sandwich between bread – no spread is needed. You could reduce the fat unit count by 2 units by using extra-light mayonnaise.

# Wholemeal pitta pockets

A wholemeal pitta bread is equally easy to take to work. Pitta pockets hold salad veg better than sandwiches – bits don't fall out. One wholemeal pitta weighs approx 50g/2oz, which is half your daily bread allowance, and supplies 3g fibre. It could be eaten along with an **F2** Essential Soup, followed by fruit, to make a more substantial meal.

Nearly all the suggested sandwich fillings could equally well be used to fill a pitta and you can freely add any salad veg. First warm your pitta bread in a toaster or under the grill to puff it up, making it easier to split open and fill. But don't leave it too long or it will go hard. Here are a few additional ideas for fillings:

## Houmous and salad

Spread the inside of the pitta with 2 rounded teaspoons reduced-fat houmous. Fill with an appropriate **F2** Essential Salad (pages 112–26), such as grated carrot with almonds and raisins, or the bean, sweetcorn, onion and red pepper mix.

## Pesto chicken salad

Mix together 1tbsp light mayonnaise with 1tsp pesto sauce, then spread inside pitta. Fill with 50g/2oz sliced cooked free-range or organic chicken breast meat, shredded lettuce, sliced tomato and cucumber.

## Cottage cheese and date

Stir a small tub of cottage cheese and chop up some dates. Spoon up to 100g/4oz of cottage cheese into the dry pitta bread and then sprinkle in the dates so that they are evenly dispersed.

## Cheese salad with salsa

Mix some tomato salsa with a few quartered cherry tomatoes, chopped yellow pepper, chopped red onion and 50g/2oz feta cheese. Add a few halved, stoned olives if you like. Pile into the pitta.

# Wholemeal pasta meals

Wholemeal pasta makes the perfect F2 meal. It is widely available in a variety of shapes – conchiglie, fusilli and spaghetti. An average (90g/3½oz dry weight) main-course serving supplies a substantial quantity of fibre, in the region of 8–9 grams. Pasta is also highly recommended for its low GI.

The obvious way to serve it as an easy meal is with the Basic Tomato Sauce on page 195, a ready-made sauce from the chart on page 147–50, or the VERY Easy Tomato Sauce on page 170. A green salad (buying a ready-to-serve pack of mixed leaves doesn't make you a bad person!) is all you need to accompany it. Raw sugar-snap peas sliced lengthways add crunch and fibre to green salad and, when you can afford the fat units, a little sliced avocado turns this salad into something really special.

If you choose the 'make in quantity and freeze' tomato sauce option, here are some of the many ways you can ring the changes. We've included 1½ fat units for a portion of the homemade tomato sauce in each meal total.

### Pasta vongole

Add 1 tbsp dry white wine and finely chopped fresh red chilli (or ½ tsp dried crushed chillies) to the tomato sauce, heat in a pan then add about 75g/3oz drained and rinsed canned baby clams and heat through gently. Stir in chopped fresh parsley.

## Calamari or seafood sauce

Add 1tbsp red wine and 1tsp garlic purée to the tomato sauce, heat in a pan then add 75g/3oz calamari (squid rings) and cook gently for 3–4 minutes until tender. For a spicy kick add chopped fresh chilli, chilli sauce, Tabasco or cayenne pepper (whatever you happen to have). Alternatively, add 75g/3oz cooked shelled prawns or seafood selection to the tomato sauce.

## Roasted vegetables

Toss a selection of thickly sliced onions, courgettes and red or yellow peppers in 1tsp olive oil in an oven-proof dish. Add crushed garlic and chopped fresh rosemary, if liked, then roast in a hot oven for 20 minutes until tender and slightly charred. Add to the tomato sauce.

## Garlic and anchovy

Add four drained and chopped anchovy fillets and 1tsp garlic purée to the tomato sauce. Just before serving, stir in a handful of shredded fresh basil leaves.

## Tuna and mushroom

Gently cook 75g/3oz sliced mushrooms in the tomato sauce, then stir in a small drained can (about 80g) of tuna in brine and 1tbsp rinsed and chopped capers.

### Veggie puttanesca

Add a good slosh of chilli sauce, 1tbsp rinsed and chopped capers, 6 chopped stoned black olives and 25g/1oz chopped sun-dried tomatoes, well drained of oil, to the tomato sauce.

## VERY Easy Tomato Sauce

Simply simmer a can of chopped tomatoes with a couple of sliced spring onions until most of the liquid has evaporated. Then add seasoning, a torn basil leaf or two, a few capers, some black olives, chopped parsley – anything you have handy. The only oil is in any olives you might use. Count 1 unit if you add 6 olives.

# Stir-fry meals

A stir-fry makes an ideal **F2** meal: loads of lightly cooked veg and only a little, if anything, in the way of animal products. Even if your chosen veg are not particularly fibre-rich, the sheer volume of veg in a stir-fry totals up to a decent quantity of fibre. And you could add high-fibre mange-tout, sugarsnap peas or baby sweetcorn which stir-fry well.

A big stir-fry can be cooked in just 2 teaspoons of olive oil in a good non-stick pan. You'll find recipes for stir-fry sauces on page 196 or you can take the fast option, selecting shop-bought low-fat stir-fry sauces from the Fat and Calorie Controller selection.

## Shop-bought option

**4 fat units for 2 tsp oil for frying (add units from chart for sauce)**

Choose any supermarket pack of ready-prepared stir-fry veg. Use the whole pack – ideally add sugarsnap peas or mange-tout for extra fibre. If you use a shop-bought stir-fry sauce add fat units from the chart.

## Homemade option

**4 fat units for 2 tsp oil for frying. Add 1 unit for Basic Stir-Fry Sauce (page 197) or choose fat-free Sweet Sour Sauce (page 198)**

Your stir-fry can be made from any mix of veg you have to hand, but should be varied for an appetizing dish. These veg are particularly good for stir-frying: roughly sliced cabbage, spring greens or pak choi, finely sliced peppers, diagonally sliced carrots, courgettes, green beans or spring onions, baby sweetcorn halved lengthways, sliced bamboo shoots (from a can), whole asparagus tips, mange-tout, sugarsnap peas, beansprouts, small broccoli florets (slice the stems so they cook quickly).

## What you could add

Stir-fried veg can be served alone or with any of the following. Just add and heat through in the final minute or two of cooking:

● **Cooked free-range chicken,** 75g/3oz of strips of skinless, boneless cooked breast meat – add 1½ fat units to meal.

● **Cashews or peanuts,** 15g/½oz are all you can afford because of their high fat content, but they will give your stir-fry a lovely crunch – add 2½ fat units to meal.

● **Cubes of firm white fish,** such as monkfish, anything up to 175g/6oz – add ½ fat unit to meal.

● **Scallops,** 75g/3oz – add ½ fat unit to meal total. Slice and stir-fry scallops for 2–3 minutes until they look opaque. Take care not to overcook or they will be tough.

● **Prawns,** 75g/3oz, peeled – add ½ fat unit to meal total. Cooked prawns should just be heated through, peeled raw tiger prawns will take a little longer – stir-fry for 2–3 minutes until they turn pink.

## Omelette meals

Eggs can team up with **F2** veg to make a fibre-rich omelette. Serve this as a main meal, with additional veg. Those who think of a cheese omelette as 'just a light lunch' can't have costed out the calories – around 550 (mainly in the form of saturated fat) even when made with a modest 40g/1½oz cheese and cooked in less than 25g/1oz of butter.

To make a much healthier lower-calorie omelette, whisk 2 Omega-3 free-range medium-sized eggs with 1tbsp milk and seasoning. Heat 1tsp vegetable oil in a non-stick frying pan (about 15–18cm/6–8inch in diameter), pour in the egg and swirl it round to cover the base. Cook on a gentle heat for 2–3 minutes, tilting the pan and drawing the cooked egg into the centre with a spatula so the uncooked mixture seeps underneath. When there's very little runny egg left, add your chosen filling, then leave the omelette undisturbed for about 30 seconds until the filling is warmed through and the omelette is golden on the base. Slide out on to a warm serving plate, flipping it in half as you do so.

Serve immediately with cooked high-fibre vegetables such as peas, sugarsnap peas or mange-tout, green beans, spinach or with 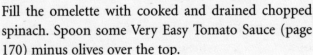 salads. Here are some simple fat-free fillings. The 6 fat units in each case are for the eggs and cooking oil.

## Mushroom omelette

You can make the filling simply by microwaving 115g/4oz sliced button or cup mushrooms in their own juices. Or add a crushed garlic clove then, after microwaving, stir in 1tsp wholegrain mustard and a sprinkling of Worcestershire sauce to make Devilled Mushrooms. Another alternative is to microwave a pack of roughly sliced mixed oyster mushrooms with ½ tsp soy sauce, 1tsp chopped fresh thyme and black pepper.

## Spinach omelette with tomato sauce

Fill the omelette with cooked and drained chopped spinach. Spoon some Very Easy Tomato Sauce (page 170) minus olives over the top.

### Leek and tomato omelette

Slice a medium-sized leek and microwave it in a bowl with the contents of a small can (230g) of chopped tomatoes with herbs. Cook on full power for 3–4 minutes or until the leeks are tender, then drain off the excess tomato juice. Fill the omelette with this mix.

### Asparagus omelette

Asparagus is a delight – the butter usually served with it a disaster. An omelette lets you enjoy asparagus without clogging arteries and gaining weight. Use about 50g/2oz asparagus tips or thin asparagus – either steam over boiling water for about 5 minutes or microwave with a splash of water in a covered dish for 2½ minutes, until just tender. Season with pepper then lay asparagus on to the omelette. For extra flavour you could add some snipped chives or chopped fresh tarragon or dill to the egg mixture.

## Baked potato meals

Bring back the baked potato! High fibre? True. High GI? Also true. But it's the low GI of a whole meal that matters. This can be sorted in several ways, by serving half a grapefruit or **F2** pulse-based soup as a starter, for instance, or serving your potato with plenty of relatively low-GI veg like peas, beans, carrots, chickpeas. It's the usual big dollop of butter that does the real damage when people eat baked potatoes. There are two ways to avoid this without too much pain.

**1** Serve your baked potato with something moist (see ideas below).

**2** Halve the baked potato lengthwise, scoop out some of the flesh and mix with one of the moist sandwich fillings on page 163–6. Count the same number of fat units for this meal and serve with an **F2** pulse-based salad.

But don't go berserk and bake yourself a boulder-sized spud. The potato is among the higher calorie veg. We'd suggest 200g/7oz maximum weight, which supplies you with 7g dietary fibre.

If you prefer to microwave your potato, wash, dry and prick it all over, sit it on kitchen paper, then cook on full power for 4–5 minutes until tender. Allow to stand in the microwave for 2–3 minutes more to ensure it cooks right through. For a crisper skin pop it in a really hot oven for 10 minutes after microwaving – an opportunity to cook other appropriate veg such as halved tomatoes at the same time.

## Baked potato, baked beans and bangers

This will help if you feel the urge (it can happen to the best of us!) to abandon all and speed off to a lorry-driver's caf. Partner your baked potato with a can of baked beans and two Quorn sausages. HP . . . tomato ketchup? By all means slosh them on. Quorn sausages, available in every supermarket, are very low in fat. Try them.

## Baked potato and ratatouille

Ideally serve with homemade ratatouille (page 201), but if you use a chilled or canned ready-made variety check with the Fat and Calorie Controller (pages 130–58) and adjust fat units if necessary. Serve with sugarsnap peas, green beans or butter beans. If you bake your potato in the oven you can also bake small halved onions or large shallots and large mushrooms. One teaspoon oil (2 extra fat units) would be enough to oil all additional veg.

## Baked potato, mushy peas and fish

Lay a 175g/6oz cod or haddock fillet in a lightly oiled dish, sprinkle with lemon juice and seasoning, then cover with foil and bake in the oven for 15 minutes (or 20–25 minutes from frozen) while you are baking your potato. Serve with a can of mushy peas (or ordinary peas if you prefer). Not quite the chip shop, but the best we can do.

## Baked potato with spicy chickpeas and crisp salad

Make a little cooking go a long way by making Spicy Chickpeas with Rich Tomato Dressing from the recipe on page 116. Serve one portion hot with a baked potato and green salad as a main meal. Allow the remainder to cool, mix in celery and sweetcorn and keep in the fridge as an Essential Stand-By Salad.

# Pizza meals

Choose a low-fat or mini pizza from our Fat and Calorie Controller. Alternatively, buy a ready-made pizza base, top with Basic Tomato Sauce (recipe on page 195) or half a jar of ready-made pizza topping, then add any of the items suggested below. Either way, serve your pizza with big heaps of **F2** Salads to turn it into a healthy fibre-rich meal.

## Home-topped pizza

● 1½ fat units for ready-made pizza base (23cm/9 inch) or 1 for a mini (14cm/5½ inch) ready-made pizza base.

● PLUS 1½ fat units for portion of homemade tomato sauce or half jar of ready-made pizza topping.

**Cheeseless Pizza Options.** Add any of the following to your pizza, calculating the appropriate number of fat units.

● Fat-free ingredients – capers, pricked small whole or halved cherry tomatoes, thinly sliced red or green peppers, sliced button mushrooms, sweetcorn, drained pineapple chunks, small broccoli florets (blanched in boiling water for 1 minute), thinly sliced onion.

● ½ fat unit – 3 halved stoned black olives.

● ½ fat unit – drained small can of tuna in brine.

● 1½ fat units – 75g/3oz cooked free-range chicken breast, shredded.

**Cheesy Options.** These toppings use just a little cheese – not the quantity that makes so many supermarket and restaurant pizzas so fattening. In each case, first spread the pizza base with tomato sauce. Add one of the following toppings, then bake in a hot oven for 10 minutes.

Fat units include tomato sauce and a 23cm/9 inch pizza base. You may prefer to use a mini-base, in which case subtract ½ a fat unit from each total.

### Spinach, tomato and ricotta

Microwave 100g/3½oz baby spinach for 1–2 minutes until just wilted. Drain and squeeze out excess water. Spread spinach in small loose heaps over the pizza, dot in between with 50g/2oz ricotta (curd) cheese, placing it in small blobs. Place 3–4 halved cherry tomatoes in between the spinach and cheese and sprinkle with freshly ground black pepper. On a mini pizza base use just 25g/1oz cheese, less veg and tomato sauce.

## Perilous pizza

**FAT** UNITS
**12**

You'll find these mega-fattening heart-stoppers in every superstore – loaded with artery-blocking saturated fat in all that cheese, often topped with processed meat to get your bad bacteria smacking their lips. A double whammy for your system! At least 1,000 calories in this and other cheesy pizzas. And at least 12 units of fat. Sometimes as many as 18. And where's the fibre?

# Permissible pizza

**FAT UNITS 3**

Even pizza can feature in healthy weight-loss when – as in all meals – you change the balance on the plate. Lots more veg, for instance bio-active **F2** salads – lots less cheese, no meat. Mini pizza, topped with tomato sauce, spinach, tomatoes and just a little ricotta, costs just 3 fat units (approx 300 calories) and you could have a larger one for 5 units. Recipes on the previous pages.

## Red pepper, feta and rocket

**FAT UNITS 5½**

Cut one roasted red pepper, drained of brine, into strips and arrange on the pizza. Scatter with 25g/1oz crumbled feta cheese and 3 stoned and halved black olives. Season with pepper. Bake, then serve garnished with rocket leaves or torn fresh basil.

## Hawaiian

**FAT UNITS 5½**

Scatter 2 tbsp sweetcorn kernels, about 75g/3oz drained pineapple chunks (half a small can) and 3 roughly chopped drained sunblush tomatoes over the pizza. Sprinkle with 25g/1oz grated mozzarella.

## Artichoke, red onion and mozzarella

**FAT UNITS 5**

Scatter 2–3 thickly sliced artichoke hearts, drained of brine (not the ones in oil), ¼ thinly sliced red onion and 1tbsp drained and rinsed capers over the pizza. Top with 50g/2oz thinly sliced 'light' or 'reduced-fat' mozzarella. If using regular mozzarella just use 25g/1oz grated.

# Meals with fish

White fish, which is very low in fat, makes a good ingredient for **F2** meals. Oily fish, much higher in fatty
calories, can be eaten in small quantities. Here are some
fishy Easy Meal ideas.

### Parcel-baked fish

Sit a chunky white fish steak (or a folded plaice fillet
for an extra half unit), on a sheet of foil and pile sliced
leeks and mushrooms on top. Season and sprinkle
with 1tbsp lemon juice. Parcel securely to seal, then
bake in an ovenproof dish at 200°C/gas 6 for 12–15
minutes. Carefully open the parcel to check that the
fish flakes easily, resealing and returning to the oven
for a further 5 minutes if necessary. Serve with peas or
sliced green beans and carrots. As this meal is so low in
fat you could also, if you wished, serve it with boiled
parsnips, mashed with a teaspoon of butter (add 1½ fat
units).

### Pesto fish with roasted veg

Chop one small red onion, one courgette and one red
pepper into chunky pieces and toss in 1tsp oil in an
ovenproof dish. Season and sprinkle with crushed
garlic. Bake at 200°C/gas 6 for 15 minutes then remove
from the oven. Brush the top of a 175g/6oz white fish
fillet with 1tsp pesto sauce and snuggle it in with the
veg, also adding some whole cherry tomatoes. Return
to the oven for 15 minutes until everything is tender.
Serve with cabbage, greens or kale.

## Smoked haddock with poached egg

Cook 175g/6oz smoked cod or haddock fillet, sprinkled with a little lemon juice and black pepper, in a covered dish in the microwave for 2–3 minutes on full power. Meanwhile poach one Omega 3, medium-sized free-range egg in a pan of simmering water. Leave the fish to stand, still covered, while microwaving 225g/8oz ready-washed young leaf spinach in its pack. What looks like a huge quantity of leaves cooks down to a small heap. Serve the fish and poached egg on the drained spinach. Grilled tomatoes make a good second veg.

## Easy-peasy paella

Make up 50g/2oz – about half a packet – of golden vegetable savoury rice (long grain rice with peas, red peppers and carrots), following the pack instructions. Add extra chopped tomatoes, diced red pepper and 115g/4oz thawed frozen peas to the rice while it is cooking. Stir in 75g/3oz cooked seafood selection, chilled or frozen variety, and heat through. Serve with a ready-made **F2** side salad.

**Note:** although brown basmati rice is generally recommended on **F2**, the generous quantity of peas in this dish will take care of fibre and GI factors.

## Baked crumbed plaice with tartare sauce

Dip up to 175g/6oz plaice or lemon sole fillet in seasoned flour, then in beaten egg, then in fresh or dried breadcrumbs. Bake with some cherry tomatoes alongside on a non-stick baking sheet at 200°C/gas 6

for 15 minutes until golden and cooked through. Serve with a wedge of lemon to squeeze over and 1tbsp tartare sauce, with canned mushy/marrow peas and baby carrots as vegetable accompaniments.

### Orange and parsley salmon

Microwave a 115g/4oz salmon steak or fillet in a covered dish on Full Power for 2–3 minutes until just tender. Top the fish with a mixture of 1tsp wholegrain mustard, 1tsp runny honey, 2tbsp orange juice and 1tsp chopped fresh parsley. Cover again and leave to stand for 1 minute. Serve with a generous portion of petits pois and baby carrots.

### Tuna with beans and salsa

Grill 115g/4oz fresh tuna steak, brushed with 1tsp olive oil for 2–3 minutes each side. Season, add a squeeze of lemon, and serve with cooked baby leaf spinach and asparagus tips. Spoon 2tbsp spicy tomato salsa over the top.

# Something simple with salads

The **F2** Salads on pages 112–19 are the backbone of this healthy dieting formula. You'll often want to make a meal of them with something simple. Shellfish is an obvious choice. Here are some other suggestions:

### Smoked trout fillet

A smoked trout fillet weighing up to 175g/6oz with horseradish sauce.

## Grilled Quorn burger

A grilled Quorn burger, with favourite relish, between your two daily slices of wholemeal bread.

## Chinese spring rolls

Two average-sized (25g/1oz) Chinese spring rolls served with sweet chilli sauce.

## Cottage cheese

Carton of reduced-fat cottage cheese.

## Stuffed vine leaves

Two ready-made stuffed vine leaves from the deli counter. Drain and wipe off surplus oil with kitchen tissue if they are in oil.

## Quorn sausages with pickle

Two cold ready-cooked Quorn sausages with the pickle of your choice.

## Stuffed taco shell

A taco shell filled with shredded lettuce, plenty of tomato salsa, and half a small 215g can of refried beans, heated in the microwave. Serve with cherry tomatoes and an **F2** Salad. Two of these stuffed taco shells with plenty of salad could turn this into a main meal.

## Sushi

Individual packs of sushi vary a little from store to store, but all are low in fat.

# 14

# SAMPLE MENUS

THE **F2** FORMULA offers great scope for choice. It's so easy to put together high-fibre, low-fat meals to suit your own taste by following the rules, selecting favourite foods from the Fat and Calorie Controller and turning to Easy Meals and Realistic Recipes for inspiration. Here are a few illustrations of the kind of daily menus you might choose.

Fibre-rich meals are very filling and you shouldn't feel hungry between meals. But if you do need a snack from time to time – in the long gap between lunch and a late dinner, for instance – choose an extra piece of fruit, a bowl of **F2** Soup or a serving of **F2** Salad. Just a small helping of these soups and salads has remarkable appetite-suppressing impact.

NOTE: In these sample menus we've kept fat lower than 10 units daily to allow for any fat in your choice of **F2** Salads, salad dressings and milk and an occasional unit-counted 'indulgence'.

# Sample menu 1

## Breakfast

- **Half a grapefruit**
- **Recommended high-fibre wheat-based cereal**
  served with soya or skimmed milk, a sliced greenish
  banana and a sprinkling of sultanas or other dried fruit

## Any time

- **One of the recommended low-fat probiotic drinks
  or yogurts**

## Lunch

- **Large bowl of F2 Soup**
- **Two slices of wholemeal toast** each spread with 2 tsp
  of low-fat houmous, topped with halved cherry
  tomatoes if you wish ........................................... **(2 units)**
- **An apple, pear or orange**

## Evening meal

- **Wholewheat pasta** with homemade tomato sauce
  (page 195) or chilled supermarket-bought Amatriciana,
  Arrabbiata or Napoletana sauce .............. **(1½–3½ units)**
- **Salads:** side-servings of a green salad and an **F2** Salad
- **Serving of vanilla ice-cream** – not Cornish or luxury –
  or of Swedish Glace, with raspberries, strawberries or
  blueberries ..................................................... **(2–2½ units)**

 **Plus any fat in
salad dressings and milk**

# Sample menu 2

## Breakfast

- **Breakfast and probiotic drink or yogurt** as in Sample Menu 1

## Lunch

- **Wholemeal pitta bread** filled with 3oz reduced-fat cottage cheese and chopped dates ........................ **(½ unit)**
- **F2 Salads,** carton-packed if taken to work
- **Two kiwi fruit, clementines or mandarins**

## Evening meal

- **F2 Soup** with large slice of wholemeal toast spread with 2 rounded teaspoons reduced-fat houmous or 1 level teaspoon olive-oil-based spread.................. **(1 unit)**
- **Large Mixed-Vegetable Stir-Fry** cooked in ........ **(4 units)** 2 tsp oil, with Basic Stir-Fry Sauce (page 197) or selected low-fat ready-made sauce ............................ **(0–1½ units)**
- **Prawns,** 3oz added to stir-fry ................................. **(½ unit)**
- **Microwaved 'Baked' Apple** with Mincemeat (page 217) ........................................................... **(0 units)**

**Plus any fat in salad dressings and milk**

# Sample menu 3

## Breakfast

- **Breakfast and probiotic drink or yogurt** as in Sample Menu 1

## Lunch

- **Sandwich** of Tuna and Sweetcorn or Tuna and Bean with light mayonnaise (see page 164) .............. **(3½ units)**
- **F2 Salad,** carton-packed if taken to work
- **Bunch of grapes**

## Evening meal

- **Cottage Pie:** homemade from recipe on page 207, or whole pack of shop-bought Quorn Cottage Pie served with peas, carrots or other fibre-rich veg ........ **(2½ units)**
- **Baked Banana** (see page 217) ............................. **(0 units)**

**Plus any fat in salad dressings and milk**

# Sample menu 4

## Breakfast
- **Breakfast and probiotic drink or yogurt** as in
  Sample Menu 1

## Lunch
- **Bowl of F2 Soup**
- **Rose Elliot's Warm Butter Bean Salad**
  (page 114) .......................................................... **(2½ units)**
- **Apple, orange or pear**

## Evening meal
- **Home-topped pizza:** spinach, tomato and ricotta on
  ready-made 23cm/9 inch base (see page 178) .... **(5 units)**
- **F2 Salads**
- **Meringue nest** topped with raspberries, strawberries
  or blueberries and a little raspberry sauce .......... **(0 units)**

**Plus any fat in
salad dressings and milk**

# Sample menu 5

## Breakfast

- **Breakfast and probiotic drink or yogurt** as in
  Sample Menu 1

## Lunch

- **Eggs:** two medium-sized free-range Omega 3 eggs,
  poached, served on two slices of wholemeal toast
  (spread, if liked, with a little mustard or
  Marmite) ............................................................ **(4 units)**
- OR **Egg, Watercress and Tomato Sandwich**
  (page 165) ........................................................ **(3½ units)**
- **F2** Salads
- **An apple or grapes**

## Evening meal

- **Bowl of F2 Soup**
- **Baked Potato with Mediterranean Ratatouille,**
  homemade from recipe on page 201 or shop-bought
  (page 154), served with green beans and
  carrots ............................................................ **(1–3 units)**
- **Simple Red Fruit Salad** (page 219) .................... **(0 units)**

**Plus any fat in
salad dressings and milk**

# Sample menu 6

## Breakfast

- **Breakfast and probiotic drink or yogurt** as in
  Sample Menu 1

## Lunch

- **Sushi:** individual shop-bought pack ............... **(1½ units)**
-  **Salads**
- **Orange or pear**

## Evening meal

- **Tomato and Red Pepper Dhal** (recipe page 203) or
  shop-bought dhal (page 141) on brown basmati rice
  with yogurt raita and mango chutney ........**(1½–3 units)**
- **Green salad** of lettuce, sliced sugarsnap peas and
  half a small avocado, sliced ............................... **(3½ units)**
- **Exotic Jade Fruit Salad** (page 219) ................... **(0 units)**

**FAT UNITS
6½–8**    **Plus any fat in
salad dressings and milk**

# Sample menu 7

## Breakfast

- **Breakfast and probiotic drink or yogurt** as in Sample Menu 1

## Lunch

- **Baked Beans** on two slices of wholemeal toast
- **Orange or Pear**

## Evening meal

- **F2** Soup
- **Smoked haddock** topped with large poached free-range Omega 3 egg served on spinach ................ **(3 units)**
- **Favourite cheese** – 1½oz (any at 3 units per oz) ............................................................. **(4½ units)**
  with an oatcake biscuit or two cream crackers ............................................................. **(1 unit)**
- **Apple**

 **Plus any fat in salad dressings and milk**

# 15

## F2
## REALISTIC
## RECIPES

IN DEVISING these recipes for The **F2** Diet, cookery expert Maggie Pannell knows you aren't planning a prestige dinner-party and it's even possible your personal maid won't be on hand today to pour your bath. Shame! So she's cut out the fuss and fiddle and come up with some healthy low-fat recipes that are really easy to make. We urge you, in particular, to make generous quantities of some of the basics, like the tomato and curry sauces and ratatouille, and freeze them in portions before you begin **F2**. You will, we promise, be very glad you did.

Following these main-meal recipes you'll find some easy, fruity desserts, providing healthy and helpful answers to sugar cravings.

**Fat units** given for each recipe are for an individual portion.

**Salt:** we've left the quantity used to you, but advise as little as possible for reasons of health.

# Basic Tomato Sauce

An indispensable and versatile tomato sauce, which can be varied with extra ingredients (see ideas below). Make up the basic sauce and freeze it in individual portion sizes, then use it as a quick pasta sauce or for a pizza topping.

## MAKES 4 PORTIONS

- 1 medium onion
- 1 medium carrot
- 1 celery stick
- 1 tbsp olive oil
- 1–2 garlic cloves (depending on the size of the cloves)
- 400g can chopped tomatoes
- 300ml/½ pint vegetable stock
- 2 tbsp tomato purée
- ½ tsp dried oregano
- pinch of sugar
- salt and freshly ground black pepper

## VARIATIONS
- 1 tbsp chopped fresh herbs, such as chives, basil or parsley.

*or*

- A pinch of chilli powder or sauce.

*or*

- 1 tbsp chopped stoned olives, capers or anchovies.

**1** Peel and chop the onion and carrot. Trim the celery and also chop it. Heat the oil in a saucepan, add the vegetables and cook them gently on a low heat for 7–8 minutes until softened but not coloured. Crush the garlic into the pan and cook for a further 2 minutes.

**2** Add the tomatoes with their juice, the stock, tomato purée, oregano and sugar. Bring to the boil then reduce the heat and cook gently for 15–20 minutes, until the vegetables are tender.

**3** Allow to cool, then tip into a blender or food processor and whizz briefly – it needn't be completely smooth. Season to taste with pepper and salt if necessary.

**4** Allow to cool completely then pack the sauce into small plastic containers ready for freezing.

**5** Thaw thoroughly, add any of the extra flavourings suggested below if liked, then use as required, either for spreading on a pizza base or reheated for serving with pasta.

**For a pasta sauce**, reheat gently with 50g/2oz sliced mushrooms, or 50g/2oz cooked prawns (½ fat unit) or 1 chopped roasted red pepper. You can buy roasted peppers in jars, packed in GI-lowering vinegar (not oil), in the supermarket. Once opened they keep well in the fridge and make a useful and convenient fat-free vegetable for adding to salads, pasta dishes, pizzas and sandwiches.

# **F2** Stir-fry sauces

Stir-fries are not only quick and easy but can be cooked in a very small quantity of oil. The fast-cooked vegetables retain their colour, bite and nutritional value. You can make them the very easy way with supermarket ready-prepared veg and sauces, or, better still, this do-it-yourself way which is still easy.

Strips of skinless and boneless chicken or turkey, chunks of firm white fish or seafood can be added to your selection of vegetables, cut up into bite-sized pieces, for a stir-fry. Or you can use vegetables alone.

Simply have all your ingredients ready to hand before you start cooking. Heat a wok or deep frying pan until it is very hot, add 2 tsp vegetable oil (4 fat units), swirl it around the pan, then when it is hot, add the food to be cooked and stir-fry by tossing it around with a spatula over a high heat and keeping it moving.

Vegetable stir-fries can be made with whatever vegetables you have to hand, but should be varied for an appetizing dish. The art is adding them to the pan in the right order so they're all cooked to perfection. Tougher vegetables go in first and delicate ones last. When the ingredients are just tender, pour over the sauce, stir-fry for a further 1–2 minutes over a high heat then serve immediately. If you use sufficient vegetables they make a meal in themselves, but a stir-fry could be served with Chinese noodles or with basmati rice.

# Basic Stir-Fry Sauce

Add fat units for oil used in frying veg, and for any meat or fish.

**MAKES 2 PORTIONS OF SAUCE** for 2 stir-fry meals, each to serve 1

- 1tbsp soy sauce
- 1tbsp dry sherry
- 1tsp honey
- 1tsp sesame oil
- 1tsp cornflour
- 6 tbsp water
- 1 garlic clove
- small piece of fresh root ginger, about 15g/½oz

**1** Measure the soy sauce, sherry, honey and sesame oil into a jug. Blend the cornflour with 1tbsp water to make a smooth paste, stir in the rest of the water then add to the sauce mixture.

**2** Peel and crush the garlic. Peel and finely chop the ginger. Add both to the sauce and stir well.

**3** Cover and keep in the fridge. If more convenient, divide between two jars.

**4** Stir before using. First stir-fry your chosen ingredients in 1–2 tsp vegetable oil, then when tender add the sauce and toss together over a high heat. Scatter with spring onions if liked.

# Sweet and Sour Sauce

Add fat units for oil used in frying veg, and for any meat or fish.

**MAKES 2 PORTIONS OF SAUCE** for 2 stir-fry meals, each to serve 1

- 1 tbsp soy sauce
- 1 tbsp cider or white wine vinegar
- 3 tbsp pineapple juice
- 2 tbsp tomato purée or ketchup
- 5 tbsp water
- 1 tbsp sugar
- small piece of fresh root ginger, about 15g/½oz
- 1 tsp chilli sauce or pinch of chilli powder (optional)

**1** Put the soy sauce, vinegar, fruit juice, tomato purée or ketchup, water and sugar in a jug. Peel and finely chop the ginger and add it to the sauce. Add chilli sauce or powder if you like a spicy kick. Stir everything well together.

**2** Keep in a jar in the fridge.

**3** Stir before using. First stir-fry your chosen ingredients in 1–2 tsp vegetable oil, then when tender add the sauce and toss together over a high heat.

# Basic Curry Sauce

Ready-made, shop-bought curry sauces, Indian ready-meals and take-aways are usually made with lots of oil. They may also include high-fat ingredients like coconut and cream. Make your own versatile, low-fat curry sauce which you can use with skinned chicken, white fish, prawns, pulses, vegetables or hard-boiled eggs to make any curry you fancy. (Add fat units for any of these ingredients used.) It's quick to make, and you can freeze individual portions, making it equally convenient to use.

## MAKES 4 PORTIONS

- 1 medium onion
- small knob of fresh root ginger, about 15g/½oz
- 2 garlic cloves
- 1tbsp vegetable oil
- 2 tbsp mild curry powder
- 400g can chopped tomatoes
- 300ml/½ pint vegetable stock
- 1tbsp mango chutney

### TO SERVE (OPTIONAL)

- 1tbsp chopped fresh coriander, per portion

**1** Peel and finely chop the onion, ginger and garlic. Heat the oil in a heavy-based saucepan, add the onion and ginger and cook gently on a low heat for about 10 minutes. Stir in the garlic and curry powder and continue to cook for 2 minutes, stirring to coat the onions evenly with the spice mixture.

**2** Stir in the tomatoes, stock and mango chutney, bring to the boil, then reduce the heat, cover and simmer gently for 15 minutes.

**3** Allow to cool, then pack into individual plastic containers, ready for freezing.

**4** When required, thaw in the fridge or defrost quickly in the microwave. Reheat gently, either in a pan or in the microwave, then add your chosen chicken, fish or vegetables (about 125g/4½oz) and simmer gently until cooked through. Stir in the fresh coriander, if liked.

**To serve** Serve your curry with boiled brown basmati rice. Allow 50g/2oz dry weight of rice and cook according to the packet instructions.

# Bolognese Sauce

Make this classic sauce for pasta with lots of vegetables and less meat for better bio-balance and less fat. It also makes a great topping for a baked jacket potato or a savoury filling for pancakes or tortillas. This recipe uses lean organic minced beef, but vegetarian meat-free mince (made from Quorn or soya protein) can be used instead. Serve the sauce on wholewheat pasta.

## MAKES 4 PORTIONS

- 1 large onion
- 1 large carrot
- 1 green pepper
- 1 large garlic clove
- 100g/3½oz sliced mushrooms
- 300g/10oz lean organic minced beef
- 400g can chopped tomatoes
- 150ml/5fl oz beef or vegetable stock, hot
- 1tsp dried oregano
- 1tbsp chopped fresh basil or parsley (optional)

**1** Peel the onion and carrot and deseed the pepper, then chop all the vegetables into small pieces. Finely chop or crush the garlic.

**2** Brown the beef in a non-stick pan for about 5 minutes on a medium heat, stirring with a spatula to break up the meat. (There's no need to add any oil to the pan if you are using beef.)

**3** Add the onion, carrot, pepper and garlic and cook gently for 5 minutes.

**4** Stir in the tomatoes, stock and oregano. Bring to the boil, then reduce the heat, cover and simmer for 20 minutes until meat and veg are cooked.

**5** Taste to check if salt or pepper is needed. Stir in the basil or parsley, if liked. Cool, then divide into 4 plastic containers. Keep chilled in the fridge or freeze.

**Cook's tip** If using Quorn or soya protein mince, first heat 1tbsp vegetable oil in the pan, then cook the mince with the onion and garlic for 5 minutes. Stir in the carrot and pepper, then the rest of the ingredients. Cook as above for 15–20 minutes.

# Mediterranean Ratatouille

FAT
UNITS
**1**

This lovely vegetable casserole, packed with sunny flavours and healthy nutrients, can make the basis for many different meals, partnering a baked potato, for instance, filling an omelette or served with grilled fish. This is such a versatile dish that if you were to make double the quantity below and freeze it in portions it would be an invaluable dieting stand-by.

**MAKES 4–5 PORTIONS**

- 1 large onion
- 1 aubergine
- 1 red pepper
- 2 medium courgettes
- 4 medium tomatoes

- 2 garlic cloves
- 1tbsp olive oil
- 2 tbsp tomato purée
- salt and freshly ground black pepper
- 2–3 tbsp chopped fresh basil (optional)

**1** First prepare all the vegetables. Roughly chop the onion, aubergine and pepper, thickly slice the courgettes, quarter the tomatoes and crush or finely chop the garlic.

**2** Heat the oil in a large flameproof casserole or heavy-based saucepan. Add the onions and cook gently on a low heat for 5 minutes, until softened. Stir in the garlic and cook for a further 2 minutes.

**3** Stir in the rest of the vegetables, cover the casserole or pan with a tight-fitting lid and cook gently for 30 minutes until the vegetables have softened. (There's no need to add any liquid as the vegetables will cook in their own juices.) Stir after 15 minutes.

**4** Add the tomato purée, season, stir then cover again and cook for a further 15–20 minutes until the vegetables are tender but not mushy.

**5** Cool, then pack into plastic tubs. Chill in the fridge, where it keeps for a couple of days, or freeze until required. Serve hot with basil.

**Cook's tip** If you'd prefer to discard the tomato skins, first blanch tomatoes in boiling water for 1 minute, then cool quickly in cold water. The skins will now slip off easily.

# Light Potato Salad

FAT
UNITS
**1**

Ready-made potato salads tend to be made with diced potato smothered with full-fat mayonnaise or salad cream. Highly fattening stuff, but not due to the much-maligned potato. The mayonnaise is the real culprit. Potatoes are among those foods which when cooked and then eaten cold become a particularly rich source of the resistant starch which is the favourite food of good bacteria. Yours will love this recipe! And since it's made with a combination of light mayonnaise and natural low-fat yogurt for the dressing, it is figure-friendly too. Use a waxy variety of potato because they hold their shape when boiled. New potatoes or those labelled as salad potatoes are ideal.

## MAKES 2 PORTIONS

- 225g/8oz baby new potatoes
- 2 tbsp natural low-fat yogurt
- 1tbsp light mayonnaise
- ½ tsp white wine or cider vinegar
- ½ tsp wholegrain mustard
- 1 garlic clove, crushed
- 2 spring onions

**1** Scrub the potatoes if not already cleaned, but do not peel them. Cut them into halves, or more pieces if large. Cook the potatoes in a saucepan of lightly salted boiling water for 10–15 minutes, until tender.

**2** Meanwhile blend together the yogurt and mayonnaise. Stir in the vinegar, mustard and garlic. Trim and finely chop the spring onions and stir them into the dressing.

**3** Drain the potatoes then stir them into the dressing. Serve warm or cold.

**Variations** Add some cooked peas to raise the fibre content and lower the GI of this dish. You could also add some finely chopped celery or gherkins to the salad, or use snipped chives in place of the spring onions.

# Tomato and Red Pepper Dhal

**FAT** UNITS **1½**

This spicy, vegetarian dhal is made with red split lentils that are really quick to cook, extremely high in fibre yet don't cause flatulence. Serve this super-healthy bio-powered dish with basmati rice and yogurt raita. For a speedy raita, stir a little mint sauce into low-fat natural yogurt and add diced cucumber.

## MAKES 4 PORTIONS

- 1 medium onion
- 2 garlic cloves
- 1 large red pepper
- 1tbsp vegetable oil
- 1tbsp curry paste (mild or medium)
- 175g/6oz red split lentils
- 400g can chopped tomatoes
- 450ml/16fl oz vegetable stock, hot
- juice of ½ lemon
- 2 tbsp chopped fresh coriander (optional)

**1** Peel and chop the onion and finely chop or crush the garlic. Cut the pepper in half, remove the seeds and white membrane then roughly chop the flesh.

**2** Heat the oil in a large saucepan, add the onion and cook gently on a low heat for 5 minutes until softened. Stir in the garlic and curry paste and cook, stirring for a further 2 minutes so that the onions are evenly coated with the spice mixture. Make sure that the heat is not too high or you could burn the curry paste and spoil the flavour.

**3** Stir in the lentils and red pepper, then add the tomatoes and stock. Bring to the boil, then reduce the heat, cover and simmer gently for 15 minutes, until the lentils are soft.

**4** Stir in lemon juice and coriander and season to taste.

**5** Allow to cool, then divide into 4 plastic containers. Keep chilled in the fridge or freeze.

**Variations** This is a very versatile dish – you can vary it by adding various extra vegetables or pulses. 150g/5oz frozen sweetcorn, peas or sliced green beans would all be good or a 400g can of drained red kidney beans. Add at the end of step 3 and heat through gently for 5–10 minutes.

# Cottage Pie

This healthy version of a popular favourite uses split lentils and plenty of veg to make a little meat go a long way. Organic beef mince is used in the recipe, but you could use Quorn for a vegetarian dish. Add the mashed potato and carrot topping to this base when you want to eat it.

### MAKES 4 PORTIONS

- 1 large onion
- 1 large carrot
- 2 celery sticks
- 300g/10oz organic lean minced beef
- 100g/3½oz red split lentils
- 500ml/18fl oz beef or vegetable stock, hot
- 1tbsp tomato purée
- 1tbsp Worcestershire sauce
- ½ tsp dried thyme
- 100g frozen peas, thawed
- 1tbsp chopped fresh parsley (optional)

### TOPPING (FOR 1 SERVING)

- 1 medium potato, about 200g/7oz
- 1 large carrot
- 2–3 tbsp milk
- salt and freshly ground black pepper

**1** Peel the onion and carrot and trim the celery, then chop into quite small pieces.

**2** Brown the beef in a non-stick pan for about 5 minutes on a medium heat, stirring with a spatula to break up the meat. (There's no need to add any oil to the pan, there's enough in the meat to prevent it from burning.)

**3** Add the onion, carrot and celery and cook gently for 5 minutes until the onion has softened.

**4** Pour in the stock and add the lentils, tomato purée, Worcestershire sauce and thyme. Bring to the boil, then reduce the heat, cover and simmer for 25–30 minutes until the meat is cooked and the lentils are tender.

**5** Add the peas and cook for a further 5 minutes. Taste to check seasoning, then stir in the parsley, if liked. Allow to cool, then divide into 4 plastic containers. Keep chilled in the fridge or freeze.

## Topping

**1** Peel the potato and carrot, cut into chunks, then cook in a pan of lightly salted boiling water until tender. Drain and mash with the milk. Season to taste.

**2** Reheat one portion of the mince mixture in the microwave, then put into a heatproof dish. Cover with the vegetable mash then put under a hot grill until crisp and golden.

# Cod with Lemon, Herb and Garlic Crust

FAT
UNITS
**1½**

Juicy courgettes and tomatoes are baked with the fish, which is then simply served with canned cannellini beans, flavoured with extra lemon and parsley.

### MAKES 2 PORTIONS

- 1 medium slice wholegrain bread, crust removed
- 1 lemon
- 2 tbsp chopped fresh parsley
- 2 garlic cloves, peeled and crushed
- 2 chunky pieces of skinless cod fillet, about 125g/4½oz each
- 1tsp wholegrain mustard
- 1tsp olive oil
- 1 large courgette, thickly sliced diagonally
- 2 firm tomatoes, halved
- freshly ground black pepper

### TO SERVE

- 300g can cannellini beans
- 1tbsp chopped fresh parsley

**1** Preheat the oven to 200°C/gas 6. Put the bread in a food processor or blender and turn into breadcrumbs. Finely grate the lemon zest and squeeze the juice. Add the lemon zest, chopped parsley and crushed garlic to the breadcrumbs, season with pepper and whizz together. Bread is quite high in salt so no extra salt is necessary.

**2** Place the fish in a lightly oiled, shallow ovenproof dish. Spread the mustard evenly over the top then sprinkle with half the lemon juice. Spoon the crumb mixture over the fish and press down lightly so that it stays in place. Drizzle with the olive oil.

**3** Arrange the courgettes and tomatoes around the fish, grind over some pepper then put the dish in the oven. Bake for 20–25 minutes, until the fish will flake easily and the topping is crisp and golden.

**4** Just before the fish is cooked, tip the cannellini beans (with their canning liquid) into a small saucepan and heat gently. When heated through, drain and toss with the remaining lemon juice, chopped parsley and pepper to season. Serve with the fish and vegetables.

**Variations** If making this dish for oneself to eat over two days, put the prepared but uncooked piece of fish on a plate, cover with cling film and keep in the fridge. Just use half the can of beans and half the vegetables. Bake the fish the following day with the vegetables as above and serve with the remaining beans.

# Tuna and Red Pepper Pizza

FAT
UNITS
2½

Add your own topping to a ready-made pizza base and you can have a tasty, low-fat alternative to the usual cheese-laden pizzas in next to no time. Serve it with an **F2** pulse-based salad and you add the vital fibre to turn this into a healthy meal. Pizza bases can be readily bought from supermarkets and you can use a portion of the Basic Tomato Sauce (see page 195) as a low-fat tasty tomato topping. Then add tuna, roasted red peppers, which can be bought in jars in supermarkets, and olives. You'll find other ideas for toppings which can be used with either homemade tomato sauce or shop-bought pizza topping sauce in the Easy Meal section on pages 176–9.

**SERVES 1 (AS A MAIN MEAL)**

- 1 shop-bought pizza base, 23cm/9 inch

- 1 portion Basic Tomato Sauce (see page 195)

- 80g can tuna in brine, drained and flaked

- 1 roasted red pepper, drained and sliced

- 4 stoned black olives, halved

- freshly ground black pepper

**1** Preheat the oven to 220°C/gas 7. Place the pizza base on a non-stick baking sheet then spread with the tomato sauce, almost to the edge.

**2** Scatter the tuna, peppers and olives over the top then season with freshly ground pepper.

**3** Bake for 10 minutes or until the base is crisp and golden. Scatter over rocket or basil leaves, if liked, and serve at once.

# Smoked Haddock Kedgeree

FAT
UNITS
2½

This well-known Anglo-Indian dish uses fragrant brown basmati rice – the best choice for fibre and GI – mildly spiced then tossed with tender flakes of smoked haddock. Traditionally it is garnished with segments of hard-boiled egg but this is not essential. A spoonful of Greek-style yogurt makes an alternative serving idea.

## SERVES 2

● 100g/3½oz brown basmati rice

● 300g/10½oz skinless smoked haddock fillet (preferably undyed)

● 1 bay leaf

● 450ml/16fl oz vegetable stock, hot

● 2 tsp vegetable oil

● 1 tsp mild curry powder

● 100g/3½oz frozen peas, thawed

● 1–2 tbsp chopped fresh parsley or chives (or 1tbsp of each)

● freshly ground black pepper

## TO SERVE (OPTIONAL)

● 1 hard-boiled egg, quartered (add 2 fat units) or 2 tbsp Greek-style yogurt (add 1 fat unit)

**1** Soak the rice in a bowl of cold water or rinse it thoroughly in a sieve to remove excess starch. This will help to keep the grains fluffy and separate.

**2** Put the haddock in a deep frying pan. Add the bay leaf, pour over the stock, then simmer gently on a low heat for 7–8 minutes, until the fish will flake easily. Remove the fish using a fish slice or a draining spoon and set aside. Pour the cooking liquid with the bay leaf into a jug and reserve.

**3** Heat the oil in the same pan, then mix in the curry powder and cook gently, stirring for about 30 seconds. Now stir in the rice until coated in the curry mixture. Pour in the reserved stock and bay leaf, bring back to the boil, then reduce the heat and cook gently for about 20 minutes until the rice is almost tender and most of the stock has been absorbed. Stir in the peas and cook for a further 3 minutes or until the rice is completely cooked and all the stock is absorbed. (Add a little extra stock if needed, before the rice is cooked.)

**4** Meanwhile, break the fish into large flakes, discarding any skin and bones. Gently stir into the cooked rice with the chopped parsley or chives, season and heat gently for about 30 seconds.

**5** Serve garnished with wedges of hard-boiled egg or a dollop of Greek-style yogurt.

# Colcannon Cakes with Poached Egg

Make up a batch of these to keep in the freezer. They can be taken out and oven baked when you want them, each served topped with a poached egg. Serve two for a main meal – just one for a light meal, reducing the fat units to 2½.

## MAKES 6 CAKES (3 SERVINGS)

- 750g/1lb 10oz floury potatoes
- 300g/11oz green cabbage or spring greens
- 3 spring onions
- 100ml/3½fl oz soya or skimmed milk

- salt and freshly ground black pepper
- 2 tbsp chopped fresh parsley (optional)

## TO SERVE

- 2 medium-sized poached eggs, or just 1 for a light meal

**1** Peel the potatoes and cut into chunks, then cook in a pan of lightly salted boiling water for 15–20 minutes until very tender.

**2** Meanwhile, finely shred the cabbage leaves, cutting out the tough stems. Put in another saucepan with just a little boiling water, or in a steamer over the potatoes. Cover and cook for about 8 minutes, until tender. Drain if cooked in water.

**3** Trim and finely chop the spring onions. Drain the potatoes thoroughly then return to the pan with the milk and mash until completely smooth. Mix in the spring onions and chopped parsley, if liked, then the cabbage.

**4** Shape into 6 thick round cakes. Open-freeze until firm, then pack into a rigid, plastic container, interleaving each cake with greaseproof paper. Use within 3 months.

## To serve

**1** Preheat the oven to 200°C/gas 6 and lightly oil a non-stick baking sheet.

**2** Put the vegetable cakes on the baking sheet, brush with a little oil and sprinkle with black pepper. Bake for 30–35 minutes until golden. Lay a poached egg on top of each to serve.

# Potato and Courgette Tortilla

FAT UNITS 6½

This famous Spanish-style flat omelette is equally delicious served hot or cold, so it makes a useful packed lunch with an **F2** Salad. Potatoes, when cooked and then eaten cold, become a source of retrograded starch which is particularly valuable for stimulating good bacterial action. This recipe includes cubes of potato and courgette and is spiced up with a little chilli, but you could add other vegetables and chopped fresh herbs to ring the changes (see variations on next page). You can buy the dried crushed chillies in a jar in the supermarket or you could add one deseeded and finely chopped fresh chilli.

**SERVES 2**

- 200g/7oz new potatoes
- 1 medium courgette
- 3–4 spring onions
- 4 medium eggs

- ½ tsp dried crushed chillies (optional)
- 1 tbsp vegetable oil
- salt and freshly ground black pepper

**1** Scrub the potatoes, then cut them into small bite-sized cubes. Add the potatoes to a saucepan of lightly salted boiling water, bring back to the boil, then reduce the heat slightly and cook gently for 5 minutes, until just tender. Drain thoroughly.

**2** Meanwhile, trim the ends from the courgette, cut it into four strips lengthways, then put the strips together and cut across the width to make small cubes. Trim and chop the spring onions.

**3** In a bowl, beat the eggs with 1tbsp cold water, add the chopped onions and dried chillies, if liked, and season with pepper.

**4** Heat the oil in a non-stick frying pan about 25cm/10 inches in diameter. Add the potatoes and courgettes and cook over a moderate heat for 10 minutes, turning and stirring from time to time, until the vegetables are light golden. Preheat the grill to high.

**5** Pour the egg mixture over the vegetables in the frying pan and cook for 3–4 minutes or until the egg has set on the base. Now place the pan under the grill and cook for a further 2 minutes to set the top.

**6** Slide the tortilla on to a plate or board and cut into wedges. Serve hot or cold.

## Variations

● To make a green-pea-and-chive tortilla, cook 150g/5oz of frozen peas in lightly salted boiling water for 2–3 minutes then drain thoroughly. Stir the peas into the beaten eggs with 2 tbsp snipped fresh chives, 1 tbsp water, and pepper to season. Pour the mixture into the frying pan and cook as from step 5 above.

● To make an asparagus and tomato tortilla, steam 200g/7oz trimmed and chopped asparagus for 5 minutes or until just tender. Stir the asparagus into the beaten eggs with 2 tbsp chopped fresh parsley, 1 tbsp water, and pepper to season. Pour the mixture into the frying pan, scatter 2 chopped tomatoes over the top then cook as from step 5.

# Spicy Bean Enchiladas

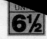

Mexican-style baked tortilla wraps with a delicious filling of red kidney beans, onion and red pepper – all superstar health veg – in a spicy tomato sauce, makes a satisfying main course served with a green salad. Passata (sieved tomatoes) is widely sold in supermarkets in cartons and jars, and flavoured with garlic and herbs makes an instant and convenient tomato sauce. You could use any canned beans, such as borlotti, pinto or haricot.

**SERVES 2 AS A MAIN COURSE**

- 1 small onion
- 1 small red pepper
- 1tbsp vegetable oil
- 420g can red kidney beans, drained and rinsed
- 500g carton passata with garlic and herbs
- ½ tsp chilli powder
- ½ tsp ground cumin
- 4 soft flour tortillas
- 30g/1oz mature Cheddar, grated

**1** Preheat the oven to 200°C/gas 6. Chop the onion and red pepper into quite small pieces.

**2** Heat the oil in a large frying pan over a low heat, add the onion and cook gently for 5 minutes until softened. Stir in the pepper and continue to cook for a further 2–3 minutes.

**3** Stir in the kidney beans and half the passata. Sprinkle over the chilli powder and cumin and bring to the boil. Reduce the heat and cook gently for 10 minutes, mashing down some of the beans with a large fork.

**4** Divide the bean filling among the tortillas, roll up like pancakes then place them side by side, seam-side down, in a shallow ovenproof dish.

...ining passata and sprinkle with the
...ne oven and bake for 15 minutes until golden
...erve hot.

**...s tip** Reseal the pack of tortillas, then refrigerate and
within 7 days, or freeze.

# Chickpea Rissoles

These little vegetarian rissoles, called falafel, are
popular all over the Middle East. Usually deep fried in
oil, in this version they are baked for a delicious low-
fat alternative. They make a great filling for pitta bread
pockets, packed out with crisp salad and a minty
yogurt dressing.

## MAKES 3 PORTIONS (12 FALAFEL)

- 410g can chickpeas, drained and rinsed
- 1 lemon
- 2 garlic cloves
- 3 spring onions
- 1tbsp olive oil
- ½ tsp ground cumin
- 2–3 tbsp chopped fresh coriander
- salt and freshly ground black pepper (or cayenne pepper)

**1** Preheat the oven to 200°C/gas 6. Line a baking sheet with greaseproof paper, unless it is non-stick in which case this won't be necessary.

**2** Grate the lemon zest and squeeze the juice from half the lemon (you'll need about 1tbsp juice). Peel and roughly chop the garlic and trim and chop the spring onions.

**3** Put the chickpeas in a blender or food processor with the lemon zest and 1tbsp juice, the chopped garlic, spring onions, olive oil, cumin and coriander. Season with salt and pepper then whizz together to make a smooth paste.

**4** Shape the mixture into 12 even-sized balls, then arrange them on the baking tray and flatten them lightly with a fork.

**5** Bake for 15–20 minutes until firm and lightly browned, turning them halfway through the cooking time. Serve warm, or cool then freeze.

**To serve** Serve four falafel in warmed wholewheat pitta bread that you have cut in half widthways and filled with crisp shredded lettuce, sliced tomato and cucumber, drizzled with a little minty yogurt dressing. To make the dressing, simply stir 1 tsp mint sauce into 3 tbsp natural low-fat yogurt. Alternatively, omit the cucumber from the salad and use tzatziki dip as a dressing.

# Honey Soy Salmon

FAT
UNITS
**6**

This meal can be ready in minutes and makes a great serving idea for salmon fillet. The salmon and mange-tout are both cooked in the microwave for speed – this also keeps the fish beautifully moist and the vegetables bright green and tender crisp. Meanwhile, all you have to do is boil some quick and easy Chinese noodles to serve as an accompaniment.

**SERVES 1**

- 1 boneless skinless salmon fillet, 100g/4oz in weight
- 2 tsp soy sauce
- 1tsp clear honey
- 1tsp wholegrain mustard

**TO SERVE**

- 50g/2oz Chinese egg noodles
- 85g/3oz mange-tout

**1** Drop the noodles into a pan of boiling water, return to the boil then simmer for 3 minutes or according to the packet instructions, until soft.

**2** Meanwhile put the salmon in an ovenproof glass dish, cover loosely with cling film, then microwave on Full Power for 2–3 minutes or just until the fish flakes easily when tested with a fork. The time will vary depending on the power of your microwave. Fish cooks very quickly in the microwave so take care not to overcook it or the flesh will be dry.

**3** While the fish and noodles are cooking, blend together the soy sauce, honey and mustard. When the fish is just cooked, remove the cling film and spoon over the soy mixture. Re-cover to keep warm.

**4** Put the mange-tout in another dish with 2 tbsp water, cover with cling film and cook on full power for 1–2 minutes until just tender. (Alternatively, they could be cooked in a steamer over the noodles.)

**5** Drain the noodles then heap them on to a serving plate. Place the salmon on top, spooning over the soy mixture. Accompany with the mange-tout.

**Variations**

If you have some spring onions in the fridge, finely shred a couple of them and scatter on top of the salmon to serve.

# **F2** Easy fruity desserts

Sweet cravings can sometimes be so strong for women that a piece of fruit doesn't quite do the trick. For those moments here are some healthy fruity desserts in which sweetness is more intense. Turn to them from time to time to stop a sweet craving turning into a binge.

## Baked apple with mincemeat

Remove the core from a large Bramley cooking apple, then run the tip of a sharp knife around the circumference to score the skin – this will stop the apple from bursting. Place the apple in a microwave-proof dish, then spoon a generous tablespoon of mincemeat into the cavity, pressing it down inside. Pour 3 tbsp apple juice into the dish then microwave on Full Power for 5 minutes, or until tender. Allow to stand for a few minutes, then serve with the juice poured over.

## Baked banana

Peel a firm banana, cut it in half widthways, then slice it again lengthways. Lay the four pieces in an oven-proof dish. Spoon over the juice of one small orange and 1tbsp maple syrup, golden syrup or honey. Bake at 180°C/gas 4 for 10 minutes until the banana is just tender and the juices are nice and syrupy. Alternatively this could be cooked for 2–3 minutes in the microwave. (This could be served with a scoop of basic vanilla-flavoured ice-cream – not luxury or Cornish – at the cost of 2 fat units.)

## Meringue with kiwi and strawberries

Mix together 2 tbsp Greek yogurt with 1 tsp lemon curd or honey then spoon into a meringue nest. (For convenience, you can buy Greek yogurt already sweetened with honey.) Top with sliced, peeled kiwi fruit and sliced strawberries.

## Peach Melba

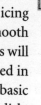

To make a quick raspberry sauce, blend 150g/5oz fresh raspberries with 2 tbsp orange juice and 2 tsp icing sugar in a blender or processor to make a smooth purée. Sieve if you prefer to remove the pips. (This will make enough sauce for 2 servings, so keep it chilled in the fridge.) Put 2 scoops of vanilla ice-cream (basic supermarket, not luxury or Cornish) into a glass dish, add one sliced ripe peach or nectarine then pour over the raspberry sauce.

**Variation** Make a strawberry sauce in the same way then pour over ice-cream and sliced fresh pineapple.

## Melon with raspberries

Cut a charentais melon in half and scoop out the seeds. (This is the variety of melon with a gorgeous fragrant peachy orange flesh.) Fill the centre of one melon half with fresh raspberries, sprinkled with just a little sugar, if liked.

## Poached pear with blueberries

Peel, quarter and remove the core from one firm dessert pear. Put the pear quarters in a pan with 100ml/3½fl oz apple juice, bring to the boil, then reduce the heat, cover and simmer for 5–7 minutes, or until the pear is almost tender. Add 50g/2oz blueberries (or blackberries) and cook gently for a further 2 minutes. Cool before eating – the pears will turn a pretty pinky-purple colour.

## Exotic jade fruit salad

Combine cubes of honeydew melon, slices of kiwi fruit and halved seedless green grapes in a serving dish. Pour over 100ml/3½fl oz apple juice or diluted elderflower cordial, then stir in a piece of finely chopped preserved stem ginger with 1tsp of the ginger syrup. You could also add some chopped fresh mint if you have some. Set aside for the flavours to mingle.

## Balsamic strawberries

This sounds bizarre, but the flavour is sensational. Slice 150g/5oz strawberries into a bowl, then sprinkle with a little caster sugar, to taste. Now sprinkle with ½ tsp balsamic vinegar and a little freshly ground black pepper. Stir gently then chill before serving. If liked serve with a scoop of fruit sorbet.

## Simple red fruit salad

Simply mix small red seedless grapes, raspberries and blueberries and keep in a bowl in the fridge. The sweetness of the grapes makes sugar unnecessary – add only a little, if any. This fruit mix is good on its own, or could be served with a little raspberry sauce (see recipe for Peach Melba), or with a low-fat ice cream, Swedish Glace (fat units on page 140) or a meringue nest.

# FURTHER READING

## Sources and References

### Dietary Carbohydrates

Cherbut, C., 'Inulin and oligofructose in the dietary fibre concept', *British Journal of Nutrition*, 2002, 87:S159–62.

Delzenne, N. M., 'Oligosaccharides: state of the art', *Proceedings of the Nutrition Society*, 2003, 62:177–82.

Food and Agriculture Organisation, 'Carbohydrates in Human Nutrition.' FAO Food and Nutrition Paper 66, Report of a Joint FAO/WHO Expert Consultation, 1998.

Food and Nutrition Board, Institute of Medicine, 'Dietary Reference Intakes for Macronutrients. Dietary Reference Intakes for Energy, Carbohydrate, Fiber, Fat, Fatty Acids, Cholesterol, Protein, and Amino Acids', National Academy of Sciences, Washington, USA, 2002.

Koh-Banerjee, P. and Rimm, E. B., 'Whole grain consumption and weight gain: a review of the epidemiological evidence, potential mechanisms and opportunities for future research', Proceedings of the Nutrition Society, 2003, 62:25–9.

Spiller, G. A. (ed.), *CRC Handbook of Dietary Fiber in Human Nutrition*, third edition, SPHERA Foundation, USA, 2001.

### Bacterial Action in the Gut

Fooks, L. J. and Gibson, G.R., 'Probiotics as modulators of the gut flora', *British Journal of Nutrition*, 2002, 88:S39–49.

Rastall, R.A., 'Bacteria in the gut: friends and foes and how to alter the balance', *Nutrition*, 2004, 134:2022S–6S.

Topping, D. L. and Clifton, P. M., 'Short-chain fatty acids and human colonic function: roles of resistant starch and nonstarch polysaccharides', *Physiology Reviews*, 2001, 81:1031–64.

### Food and the Colon

Adolfsson, O., Meydani, S. N. and Russell, R. M., 'Yogurt and gut function', *American Journal of Clinical Nutrition*, 2004, 80:245–56.

Cummings, J. H. and Macfarlane, G. T., 'Gastrointestinal effects of prebiotics', *British Journal of Nutrition*, 2002, 87:S145–51.

### Colonic Function

Cummings, J. H., Antoine, J. M., Azpiroz, F., Bourdet-Sicard, R., Brandtzaeg, P., Calder, P. C., Gibson, G. R., Guarner, F., Isolauri, E., Pannemans, D., Shortt, C., Tuijtelaars, S. and Watzl, B., 'PASSCLAIM – gut health and immunity', *European Journal of Nutrition*, 2004, 43:II118–73.

Lewis, S. J. and Heaton, K. W., 'The metabolic consequences of slow colonic transit', *American Journal of Gastroenterology*, 1999, 94:2010–6.

Muller-Lissner, S. A., Kamm, M. A., Scarpignato, C. and Wald, A., 'Myths and misconceptions about chronic constipation', *American Journal of Gastroenterology*, 2005, 100:232–42.

Scheppach, W., Bingham, S., Boutron-Ruault, M. C., Gerhardsson de Verdier, M., Moreno, V., Nagengast, F. M., Reifen, R., Riboli, E., Seitz, H. K. and Wahrendorf, J., 'WHO consensus statement on the role of nutrition in colorectal cancer', *European Journal of Cancer Prevention*, 1999, 8:57–62.

## Colon Cancer Risk

Bingham, S. and Riboli, E., 'Diet and cancer – the European prospective investigation into cancer and nutrition', *Nature Reviews Cancer*, 2004, 4:206–15.

Bingham, S. A., Day, N. E., Luben, R., Ferrari, P., Slimani, N., Norat, T., Clavel-Chapelon, F., Kesse, E., Nieters, A., Boeing, H., Tjonneland, A., Overvad, K., Martinez, C., Dorronsoro, M., Gonzalez, C. A., Key, T. J., Trichopoulou, A., Naska, A., Vineis, P., Tumino, R., Krogh, V., Bueno-de-Mesquita, H. B., Peeters, P. H., Berglund, G., Hallmans, G., Lund, E., Skeie, G., Kaaks, R. and Riboli, E., 'European Prospective Investigation into Cancer and Nutrition. Dietary fibre in food and protection against colorectal cancer in the European Prospective Investigation into Cancer and Nutrition (EPIC): an

observational study', *Lancet*, 2003, 361:1496–501.

Lupton, J. R., 'Microbial degradation products influence colon cancer risk: the butyrate controversy', *Journal of Nutrition*, 2004, 134:479–82.

## Carbohydrate Cravings and the Menstrual Cycle

Cross, G. B., Marley, J., Miles, H. and Willson, K., 'Changes in nutrient intake during the menstrual cycle of overweight women with premenstrual syndrome', *British Journal of Nutrition*, 2001, 85:475–82.

Dye, L. and Blundell, J. E., 'Menstrual cycle and appetite control: implications for weight regulation', *Human Reproduction*, 1997, 12: 1142–51.

## Glycaemic Index

Augustin, L. S., Franceschi, S., Jenkins, D. J., Kendall, C. W. and La Vecchia, C., 'Glycemic index in chronic disease: a review', *European Journal of Clinical Nutrition*, 2002, 56:1049–71.

Brand-Miller, J. C., Holt, S. H., Pawlak, D. B. and McMillan, J., 'Glycemic index and obesity', *American Journal of Clinical Nutrition*, 2002, 76:281S–5S.

Cordain, L., Eaton, S. B., Sebastian, A., Mann, N., Lindeberg, S., Watkins, B. A., O'Keefe, J. H. and Brand-Miller, J., 'Origins and evolution of the Western diet: health implications for the 21st century', *American Journal of Clinical Nutrition*, 2005, 81:341–54.

# INDEX